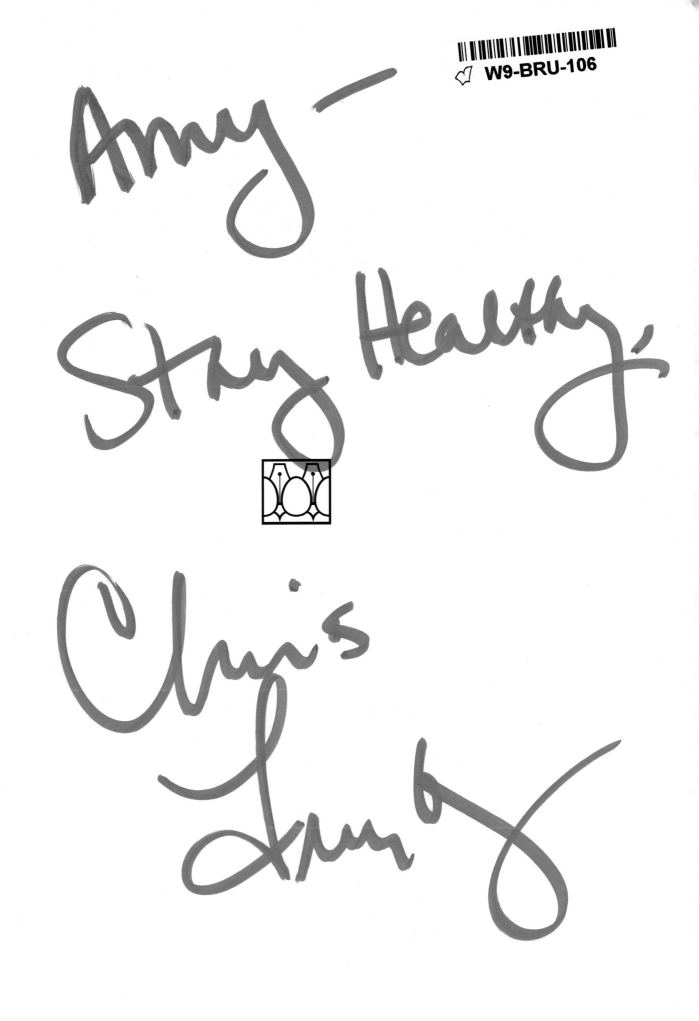

Amy —

Stay Healthy,

Chris

CHOOSE THIS!

DELICIOUS RECIPES MADE FROM SIMPLE AND NUTRITIOUS INGREDIENTS

Chris Freytag

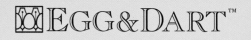

EGG&DART™

Published by Egg & Dart™, a division of Dynamic Housewares Inc

10 9 8 7 6 5 4 3 2 1

First paperback edition 2011

This book is not intended as a medical manual. It is not intended to replace personalized nutritional council. You should consult a doctor/nutritionist/personal trainer before making any drastic changes in diet or physical activity.

Author:

Chris Freytag

Book Design, Food Photographs, and Illustrations:

Christian and Elise Stella

Copy Editor:

Kelly Machamer

Manufactured in the USA

ISBN 978-0-9841887-8-9

CONTENTS

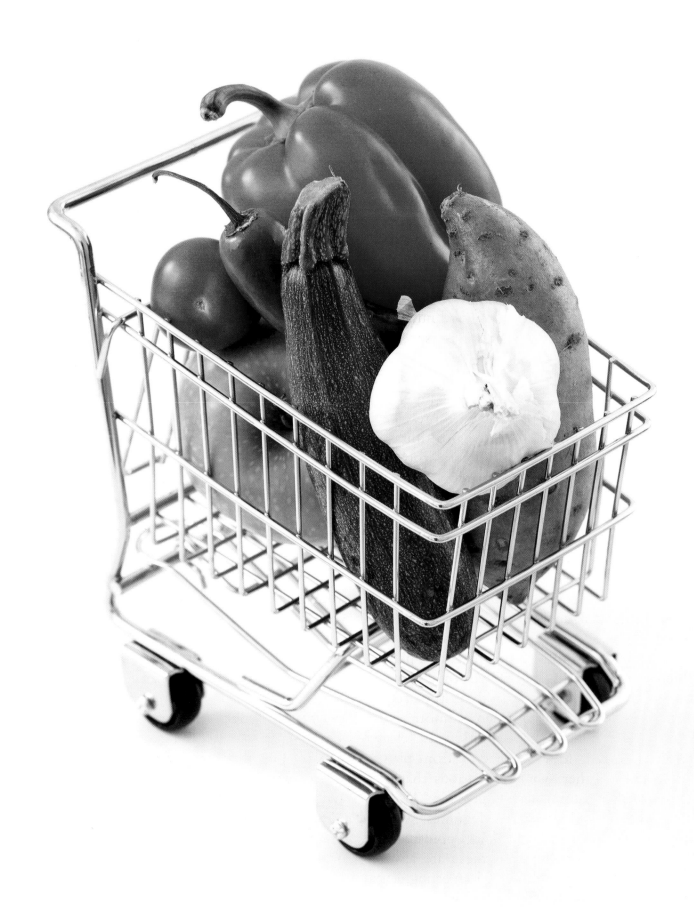

MAKING MEANINGFUL FOOD CHOICES ....

Life is about choices. We make choices every day; some are good and some are bad. When it comes to weight and overall health, a few small choices can really add up. You may not realize it, but making a few minor adjustments to the way you cook and eat could start you on a whole new path to better health.

Being a health and fitness expert, as well as a mother of 3 teenagers, I've always felt a responsibility to share my knowledge of good nutrition and healthy habits with other people, especially those with families.

I have always cooked delicious, nutritious food for my family, but it has taken many years to build up the collection of recipes presented in this book. Until recently, I did not think of my family meals as recipes. I've always thought that as soon as you know what healthy foods to cook and how to cook them, you'll have all the tools you need to create an infinite number of delicious dishes completely off the cuff. While I still believe this wholeheartedly and I still spend a lot of my time in the kitchen improvising with whichever fresh ingredients I have on hand, the recipes in this book are the ones that I always fall back on. These are the recipes I prepare when I need to prepare a healthy family meal in a pinch. (Which seems like ALL THE TIME these days!)

My recipes are about clean and healthy eating, which is something that I've been promoting for the last two decades. My definition of "clean eating" is choosing foods that come from plants or animals—in other words, real foods that are as close to their natural state as possible. Things like fresh fruits and vegetables, legumes, whole grains, low-fat dairy and lean meats, poultry, and fish. When grocery shopping, these are always the best ingredients to choose. Clean eating, at its core, is about making mindful and meaningful food choices.

Every recipe in this book features one ingredient that is highlighted and explained in a little better detail. I truly believe that education is a key component to any healthy lifestyle. Once you know exactly why a particular ingredient is good for your body, you're more likely to cook with it on a regular basis. It is my hope that this, coupled with a delicious recipe that shows a healthy technique for preparing that ingredient, will arm you with the knowledge and skills to make clean eating second nature for you and your family, as it is for me and mine. We must all eat better to live better.

Please keep in mind that striving for perfection usually leads to disaster. I have my own personal struggles with food choices from time to time, and I'll admit that I occasionally indulge in a dessert at a fancy restaurant! But the key word for any indulgence is "occasionally!" On a daily basis, I try to make food choices for myself and my family that are wholesome, healthy, nutritious, and delicious. I also find that making realistic choices will get you farther than not. While I believe that cooking something like beans from scratch—starting with the dry beans—is more natural and something I should advocate, I am realistic enough to know that most people do not have the time to do that… I know I don't! Cooking with canned beans or frozen vegetables can definitely be a part of a clean eating lifestyle. They are still a better choice for your body than unnatural overly-processed foods.

I hope you find my recipes as quick, effortless, and delicious as I do. I genuinely hope that some of the ideas I present in them can inspire you to make or continue making better choices for your own family meals.

Chris Freytag

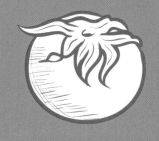

SMART STARTERS

· ·

"These recipes are proof that an appetizer doesn't have to have more calories and fat than you should be eating in an entire day!"

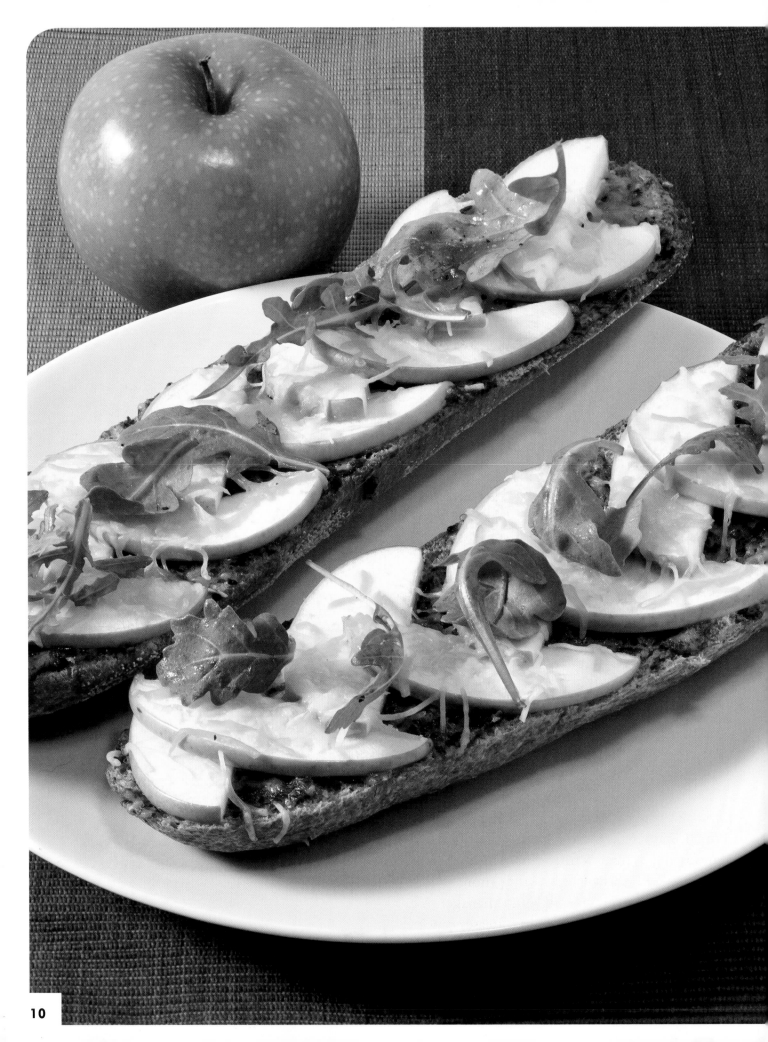

APPLE PESTO PIZZA BREAD

"This Apple Pesto Pizza Bread is a quick and easy yet refined appetizer that is topped with a creamy pesto spread, sweet apples, and peppery arugula for a little bite."

YOU WILL NEED

1 whole grain baguette

¼ cup prepared pesto sauce

1 Granny Smith apple, cored and thinly sliced

½ cup shredded Cheddar-jack cheese

1 cup fresh arugula (may use fresh baby spinach)

2 teaspoons olive oil

⅛ teaspoon salt

⅛ teaspoon pepper

CHOOSE THIS!

Whole Grains, like those in the whole grain baguette in this recipe, are much higher in vitamins, minerals, fiber, and antioxidants than refined or "white" grains. Studies have shown that eating more whole grains may help with weight management and reduce the risk of heart disease, cancer, and diabetes.

1 Preheat oven to 350 degrees F. Slice baguette in half lengthwise, separating into two long pieces.

2 Lightly spread each half of the baguette with the prepared pesto sauce.

3 Top each half with an equal amount of the sliced apple and shredded Cheddar-jack cheese.

4 Place halves on a sheet pan and bake 10 minutes, or until cheese is melted and bubbly.

5 In a mixing bowl, toss arugula in the olive oil, salt, and pepper to very lightly dress.

6 Slice the baked pizza bread into 8 equal pieces and serve topped with a pinch of the dressed arugula.

SMART STARTERS

CREAMY AVOCADO SALSA

"This Creamy Avocado Salsa is like a wonderful and nutritious combination of salsa, guacamole, and sour cream. I guess you can call it an all-in-one 3-layer dip."

YOU WILL NEED

1 cup nonfat plain Greek yogurt, drained of excess liquid

1 avocado, diced

¼ cup diced red onion

2 Roma tomatoes, diced and drained of excess liquid

1 jalapeño pepper, finely minced

¼ cup fresh cilantro, chopped

1 teaspoon lime juice

½ teaspoon cumin

½ teaspoon salt

1 In a mixing bowl, combine all ingredients, stirring to combine.

2 Cover and refrigerate for at least 1 hour to let the flavors combine.

3 Serve with vegetables, baked pita chips, or multi-grain tortilla chips.

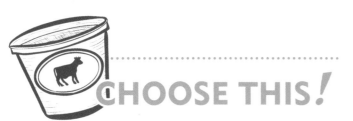

CHOOSE THIS!

Greek Yogurt is becoming more and more popular in America, and for good reason! Not only is Greek yogurt far thicker than regular yogurt, but it is also far more concentrated with protein and probiotics that can soothe and strengthen our digestive tract.

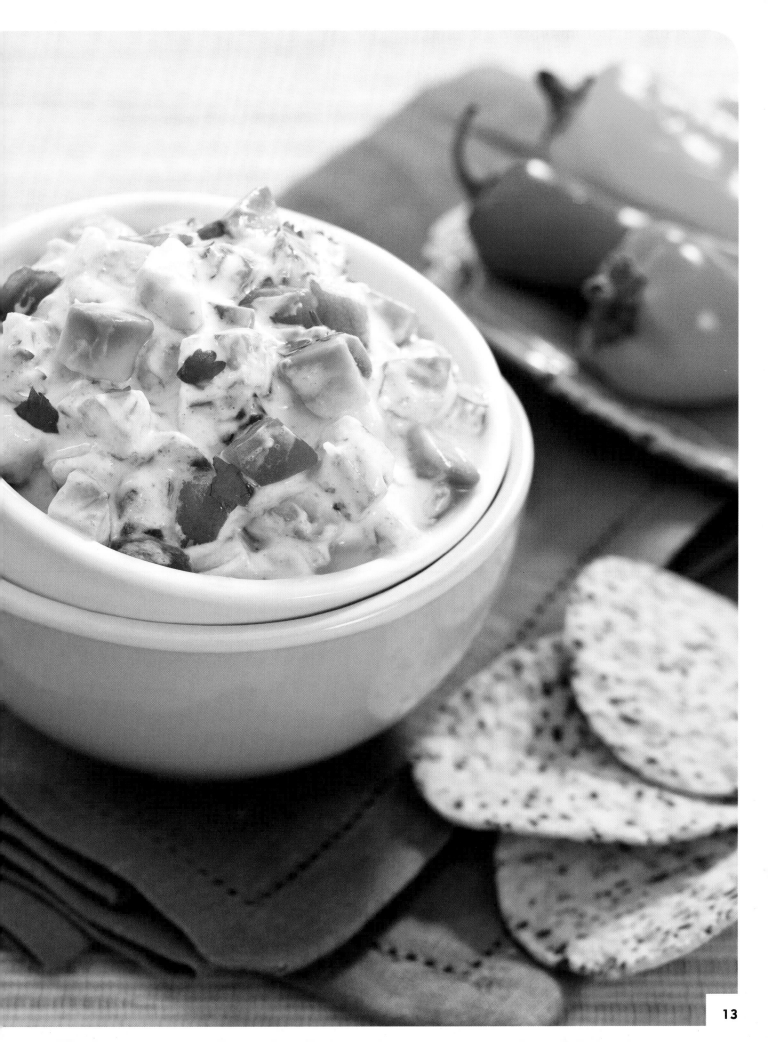

CALORIES	FAT	PROTEIN	CARBS	FIBER
110	6g	5.5g	12g	5g

ASPARAGUS WITH HOT WASABI DIP

"This recipe for blanched asparagus with a hot and spicy Asian wasabi dip makes an attractive and healthy party appetizer. While this makes a crowd's worth, you can simply halve the recipe to prepare 3 servings for snacks."

YOU WILL NEED

2-3 pounds asparagus

1 cup light mayonnaise

1 tablespoon low-sodium soy sauce

1 ½ teaspoons light agave nectar (may use honey)

2 teaspoons lemon juice

2 teaspoons wasabi paste

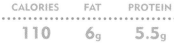

CHOOSE THIS!

Asparagus is just barely boiled (blanched) in this recipe to retain its fresh crispness and beautiful green color. Blanching also helps retain some of the asparagus' key nutrients, such as folate, vitamin C, and potassium.

1 Trim about 1 ½ inches from the stalks of the asparagus and then drop into boiling water to blanch, cooking for just 1-2 minutes. (1 minute for pencil-thin asparagus or 2 minutes for thicker asparagus.)

2 Remove asparagus from boiling water, transferring to a large bowl of ice water to stop the cooking process. Once cooled, remove asparagus from water bath and chill until ready to serve.

3 In a mixing bowl, combine all remaining ingredients to create the Hot Wasabi Dip. Cover and refrigerate for at least 30 minutes to let the flavors combine before serving alongside the blanched asparagus for dipping.

BUFFALO CHICKEN KABOBS

"These great party-friendly kabobs are healthier than traditional buffalo chicken wings in as many as three ways: they're made with white meat chicken in place of the higher-fat dark meat of the wings, they're baked instead of deep fried, and they're tossed in a lower-fat wing sauce."

YOU WILL NEED

bamboo skewers, soaked in water for 30 minutes

1 pound chicken breast tenders

¼ cup Louisiana hot sauce

3 tablespoons light butter, melted

⅛ teaspoon salt

2 stalks celery, cut into 1 inch lengths

½ cup light blue cheese dressing

CHOOSE THIS!

White Meat Chicken is much lower in fat and cholesterol than the skin and dark meat you would get in a typical buffalo chicken wing. Using chicken breast tenders in this recipe ensures that the meat is still moist and delicious.

1 Preheat broiler to high. Line a sheet pan with aluminum foil.

2 Place chicken tenders in a large bowl and cover with hot sauce, melted butter, and salt. Toss all to fully coat.

3 Thread each coated chicken tender onto 1 pre-soaked skewer and then place onto the lined sheet pan.

4 Drizzle any remaining sauce over top all kabobs and broil for about 6 minutes, flipping halfway through. Cut into one kabob to ensure that chicken is mostly white throughout.

5 Serve alongside celery and blue cheese dressing to cool down the palate.

SMART STARTERS

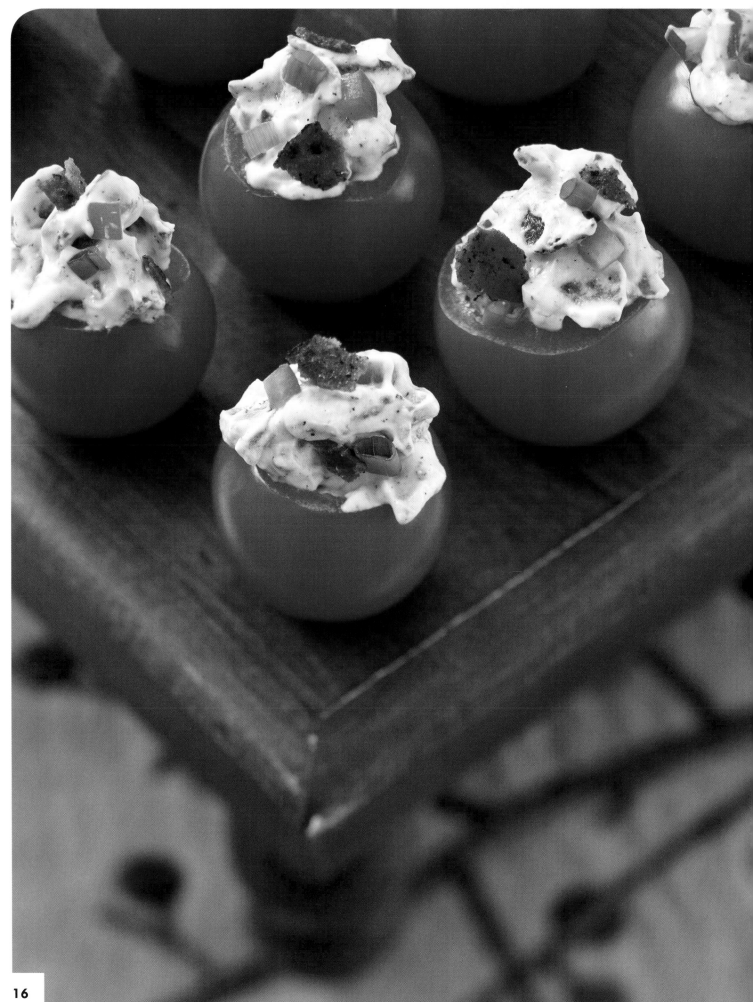

BACON STUFFED CHERRY TOMATOES

"These one (or maybe two) bite tomatoes are stuffed with a creamy bacon filling that is made from turkey bacon to dramatically cut down on calories and saturated fat. Each 80 calorie serving includes 4 generous pieces."

YOU WILL NEED

12 slices turkey bacon

½ cup fat-free sour cream

¼ cup chopped green onions

2 tablespoons minced red bell pepper

1 teaspoon Dijon mustard

¼ teaspoon honey

⅛ teaspoon salt

⅛ teaspoon pepper

2 pints cherry tomatoes (about 24)

CHOOSE THIS!

Turkey Bacon can make a great substitution for regular bacon in a recipe such as this one. It is very important that you check the nutritional labels, as some turkey bacon can be nearly as high in fat as the regular stuff! I know that Butterball is a very good choice with only 2.5 grams of fat per 2 slices.

1 Place turkey bacon in a skillet over medium-high heat and cook until thoroughly browned on both sides. Transfer browned bacon to a cutting board and let cool before finely dicing.

2 In a mixing bowl, combine sour cream, turkey bacon, green onions, red bell pepper, Dijon mustard, honey, salt, and pepper, and fold all together to create the bacon filling.

3 Slice tops off cherry tomatoes and use a melon-baller or grapefruit spoon to scoop out the seeds and membranes of each.

4 Fill each tomato with an equal amount of the bacon filling and serve at room temperature or chilled.

SMART STARTERS

PREP TIME	COOK TIME	SERVES		CALORIES	FAT	PROTEIN	CARBS	FIBER
15 mins	10 mins	8		160	9.5g	8g	9g	5g

SOUTHWESTERN SWEET PEPPER NACHOS

"These smothered nachos are actually made with sweet and crunchy red bell pepper pieces in place of high-calorie and high-fat tortilla chips."

YOU WILL NEED

6 red bell peppers

8 ounces pepper-jack cheese, shredded

½ (15-ounce) can black beans, drained and rinsed

½ cup frozen corn kernels, thawed

½ cup fresh salsa

4 green onions, thinly sliced

fat-free sour cream, if desired

1 Preheat broiler to high. Slice bell peppers into bite-sized pieces, discarding stems and seeds.

2 Spread the cut bell peppers across a large sheet pan and cover with ½ of the pepper-jack cheese.

3 Place sheet pan under broiler and broil until cheese is melted, about 2 minutes.

4 Top with black beans, corn, and all remaining cheese, and return to the broiler to melt the second layer of cheese. Cook until cheese is completely melted and the edges of the peppers are beginning to brown, about 3 minutes.

5 Remove from oven and sprinkle with the sliced green onions before serving alongside salsa, for dipping. You may also serve with fat-free sour cream, if desired.

CHOOSE THIS!

Red Bell Peppers make a sweet and crisp substitution for tortilla chips in this recipe, saving a ton of calories and drastically boosting nutrition at the same time. Bell peppers are loaded with vitamins A and C and several phytochemicals that can help protect cells from damage.

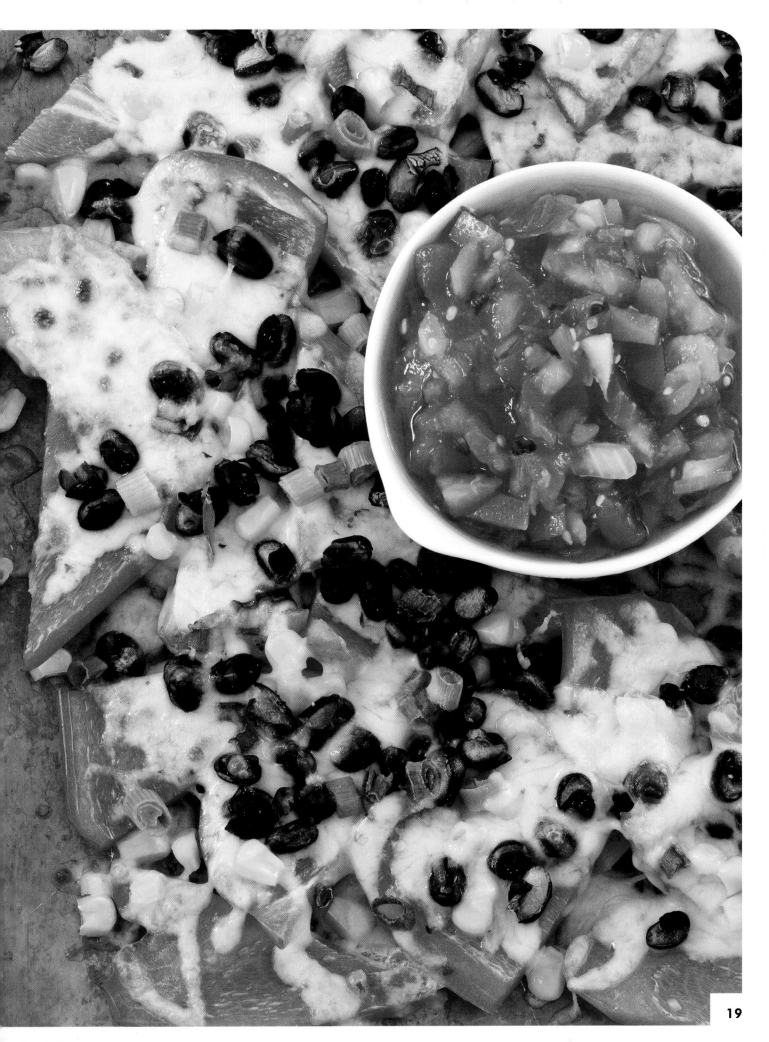

ITALIAN WHITE BEAN DIP

"This thick and creamy Italian White Bean Dip makes a delicious alternative to high-fat ranch or French-onion vegetable dips."

YOU WILL NEED

1 (15-ounce) can cannellini beans, drained and rinsed

¼ cup fresh parsley

2 cloves garlic, peeled

2 tablespoons lemon juice

1 tablespoon olive oil

2 tablespoons water

⅛ teaspoon ground red pepper

salt and pepper to taste

carrots, celery sticks, or pita chips, for dipping

1 Place all ingredients into a food processor or blender.

2 Pulse or blend until almost entirely smooth, about 1-2 minutes. Garlic cloves should be very finely chopped.

3 Season with salt and pepper to taste.

4 Serve with carrots, celery sticks, or baked pita chips for dipping. Or try serving with grilled whole wheat pitas!

CHOOSE THIS!

Cannellini Beans are not just savory and versatile, but also packed with protein and fiber to keep you feeling full and satisfied. A single serving of cannellini beans can also provide 20% of your daily recommended value of magnesium, iron, and folate.

PREP TIME	COOK TIME	SERVES
30 mins	10 mins	6

CALORIES	FAT	PROTEIN	CARBS	FIBER
350	20g	27g	22g	3.5g

ASIAN CHICKEN KABOBS

"This recipe not only makes 12 packed skewers of grilled chicken in an Asian peanut marinade but also 6 grilled vegetable skewers to serve alongside them."

YOU WILL NEED

18 bamboo skewers, soaked in water for 30 minutes
1 tablespoon ground coriander
1 onion, quartered
2 cloves garlic, peeled
½ cup low-sodium soy sauce
¼ cup lime juice
½ cup natural peanut butter
¼ cup light brown sugar
½ cup canola oil
4 boneless, skinless chicken breasts
1 onion, quartered and separated
1 red bell pepper, cut into 1-inch pieces
18 mushrooms
1 yellow bell pepper, cut into 1-inch pieces

CHOOSE THIS!

Low-Sodium Soy Sauce

can be a great way to enjoy Asian flavors with about 50% less salt content than the regular sauce. Because sodium attracts and holds water, it can actually increase blood volume, putting strain on your heart if you consume more than your kidneys can excrete.

1 In the bowl of a food processor, combine coriander, the first onion, garlic, soy sauce, lime juice, peanut butter, brown sugar, and canola oil. Process until everything is finely chopped to create a marinade.

2 Cut chicken breasts into 1-inch cubes and place in a food storage container with ¾ of the marinade. Cover and refrigerate for at least 30 minutes. Reserve remaining marinade.

3 Thread vegetables onto soaked skewers, alternating between the onion, red bell pepper, mushrooms, and yellow bell pepper. Create 6 full skewers with 3 pieces of each vegetable on each. Brush vegetable skewers with the remaining ¼ of the marinade.

4 Remove cubed chicken from marinade and thread chunks onto 12 skewers (separate from the vegetables).

5 Lightly oil a grill, indoor grill, or grill pan and set to medium-high heat. Place the vegetable and chicken skewers on grill and grill for 8-12 minutes, turning as each side browns, until chicken is entirely cooked throughout and vegetables are tender. Serve 2 chicken skewers and 1 vegetable skewer together.

SMART STARTERS

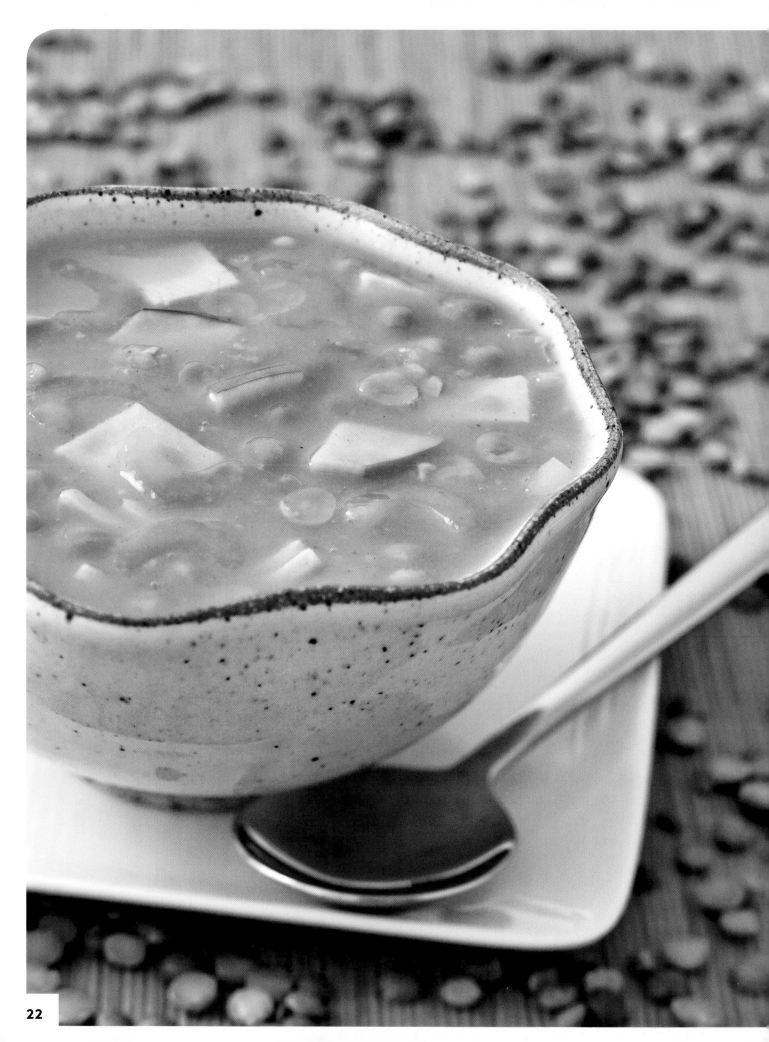

SPLIT PEA SOUP

"I believe that bacon or ham is the key to a comforting bowl of split pea soup. This recipe uses Canadian bacon to nutritiously adhere to that simple guideline."

YOU WILL NEED

1 tablespoon olive oil

1 yellow onion, chopped

½ cup chopped celery

3 cloves garlic, minced

4 cups water

5 cups reduced-sodium chicken broth

2 cups dried split peas

½ teaspoon dry marjoram

¼ teaspoon dried thyme

6 ounces Canadian bacon, diced

salt and pepper to taste

1 Heat olive oil in a large pot over medium-high heat.

2 Add onion and celery to the hot pan and sauté until vegetables have softened. Add garlic and sauté 1 additional minute.

3 Add all remaining ingredients, except Canadian bacon, and bring up to a boil. Reduce heat to low and let simmer 1 hour and 15 minutes.

4 Purée the soup using a hand held blender or cool slightly before transferring to a regular blender or food processor to blend in batches. Return soup to the stove.

5 Add Canadian bacon to the soup and bring back up to a simmer before seasoning with salt and pepper to taste. Serve hot.

CHOOSE THIS!

Canadian Bacon has about ¼ the calories and ⅓ the saturated fat of regular bacon. Choosing delicious Canadian bacon, or even low-fat turkey bacon, is just one of those easy ways that you can change bad eating habits into good ones.

SMART STARTERS

TOMATO BASIL SOUP

"This creamy tomato soup is sure to bring warmth and satisfaction to your table with an all-day taste that's made in only 30 minutes time."

YOU WILL NEED

2 (28-ounce) cans diced tomatoes

4 cups low-sodium V8 vegetable juice

1 tablespoon hot sauce

12 leaves fresh basil, chopped

1 cup low-fat evaporated milk

4 ounces fat-free cream cheese

⅛ teaspoon garlic powder

salt and pepper

CHOOSE THIS!

Low-fat Evaporated Milk

gives this soup a creamy flavor with only about ¼ of the calories of heavy cream. Evaporated milk has about ½ of the water content of milk removed, leaving you with the pure, creamy essence of dairy, which is unlike cream that gets its creaminess from fat. Be careful not to purchase sweetened condensed milk (a sugar overload!) by accident, because it is definitely NOT the same thing.

1 In a large pot, bring diced tomatoes, vegetable juice, hot sauce, and basil up to a boil. Reduce heat to medium and let simmer rapidly for 30 minutes.

2 Purée the cooked tomato mixture using a hand held blender or cool slightly before transferring to a regular blender or food processor to blend in batches. Return soup to the heat.

3 Add evaporated milk and cream cheese, and stir until all of the cheese has been incorporated into the soup.

4 Season with garlic powder and salt and pepper to taste. Serve hot alongside whole grain bread or topped with whole grain croutons.

SPICY PEANUT DIP

"This Asian-style peanut dip is not just savory, but also pretty darn spicy. The cold crunch of the celery sticks dipped into it is just the ticket to cool things down."

YOU WILL NEED

1 cup natural peanut butter

6 green onions, thinly sliced

½ cup loosely packed cilantro leaves, chopped

2 serrano chili peppers, chopped

1 tablespoon low-sodium soy sauce

juice and zest of 2 limes

1 teaspoon turmeric

carrots and celery sticks, for dipping

1 Place all ingredients into a food processor or blender.

2 Pulse or blend until almost entirely smooth, about 1-2 minutes. Peppers should be very finely chopped.

3 This dip should be very thick but can be thinned out with a few teaspoons of hot water, if desired. Add the water 1 teaspoon at a time, just until it is as thin as you want it.

4 Serve with carrots and celery sticks for dipping.

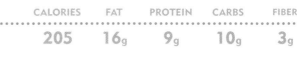

CHOOSE THIS!

Peanuts (and the peanut butter used in this recipe) are a great source of mono-unsaturated fat and other nutrients shown to promote heart health. Natural peanut butter is best because it does not contain the added sugar, corn syrup, or oil that regular peanut butter can contain.

SMART STARTERS

PREP TIME	COOK TIME	SERVES		CALORIES	FAT	PROTEIN	CARBS	FIBER
15 mins	30 mins	8		235	4.5g	10g	42g	10.5g

PUMPKIN BLACK BEAN SOUP

"Pumpkin and black beans may not seem like the perfect match, but this soup will definitely prove otherwise. Savor it on winter's coldest days."

YOU WILL NEED

2 tablespoons olive oil

1 yellow onion, diced

¾ cup diced celery

¾ cup diced carrots

3 cloves garlic, minced

1 cup red wine

3 (15-ounce) cans black beans, drained and rinsed

1 (15-ounce) can pumpkin

1 (15-ounce) can diced tomatoes

4 cups low-sodium vegetable broth

1 tablespoon ground cumin

1 tablespoon hot sauce

salt and pepper to taste

1 Heat olive oil in a large pot over medium-high heat.

2 Add onion, celery, and carrots to the hot pan and sauté until vegetables have softened. Add garlic and sauté 1 additional minute.

3 Pour red wine over vegetables in the pot and let simmer until the wine has reduced by about half.

4 Add all remaining ingredients and bring up to a boil. Reduce heat to low and let simmer 25 minutes.

5 Season with salt and pepper to taste and serve hot. For a smoother consistency: purée the finished soup using a hand-held blender or cool slightly before transferring to a regular blender in small batches. Return to the heat and bring back up to a simmer before serving.

CHOOSE THIS!

Pumpkin is extremely high in antioxidants and beta-carotene, which can help regenerate cells in the body. This effect makes it a great "age reversing" food. Its smooth and thick consistency is a great way to naturally thicken dishes like this soup.

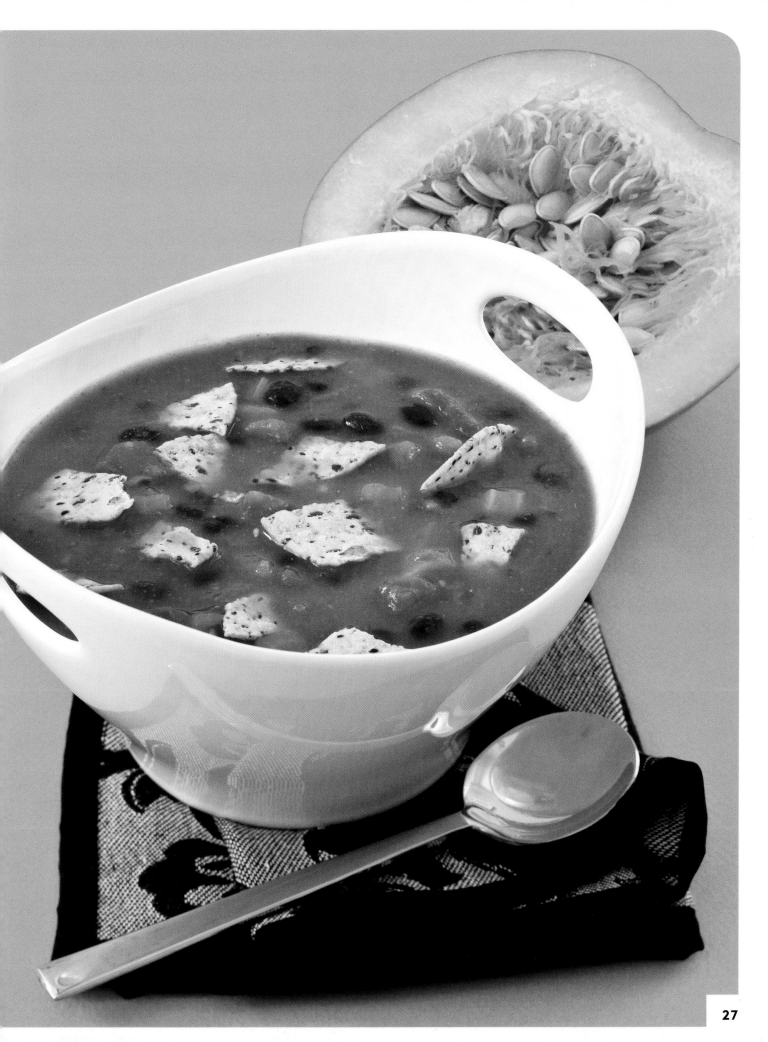

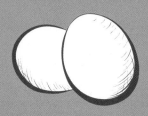

BOREDOM BUSTING BREAKFASTS

....

"Breakfast is the foundation upon which your body builds the day. You'll be surprised how good and alert you feel when you start your day with the proper fuel."

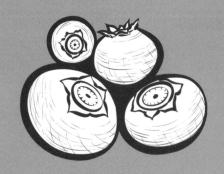

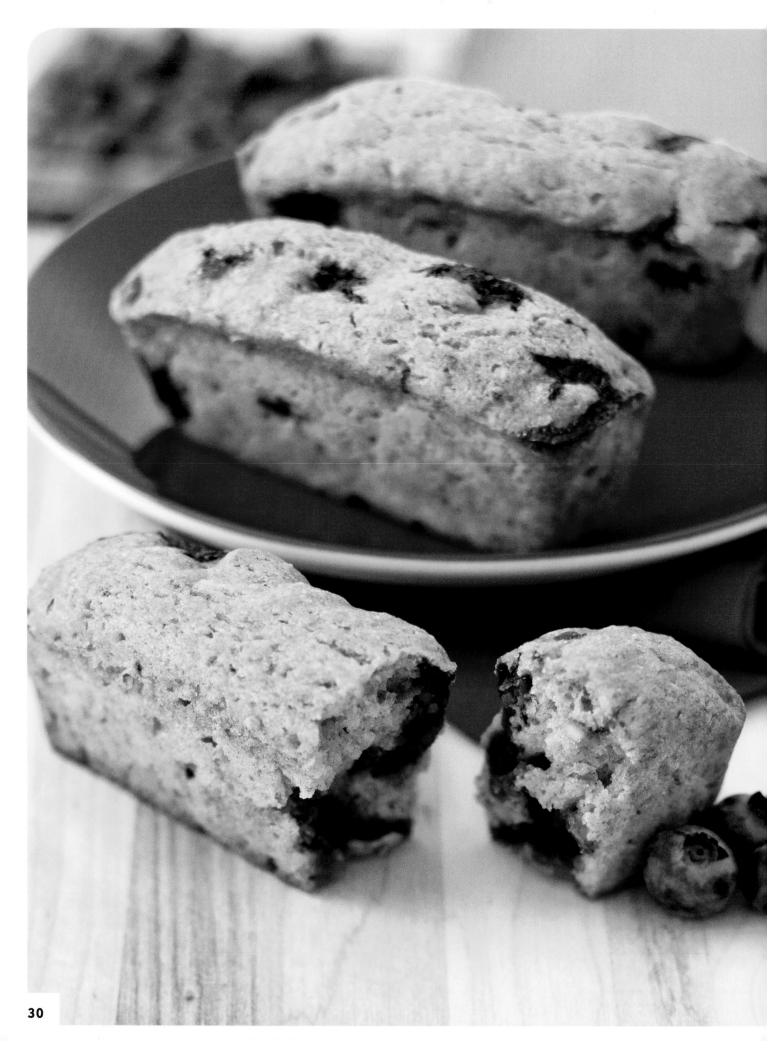

PREP TIME	COOK TIME	SERVES		CALORIES	FAT	PROTEIN	CARBS	FIBER
25 mins	40 mins	24		145	1g	3g	32.5g	2g

BLUEBERRY AND ZUCCHINI BARS

"These delicious breakfast bars are not only packed with antioxidant-rich blueberries but also nutritious zucchini that bulks them up without adding any unusual flavor. Simply grate the zucchini using a cheese grater for the best texture."

YOU WILL NEED

nonstick cooking spray
1 large egg white
1 cup apple sauce
1 tablespoon vanilla extract
2 cups sugar
2 cups all-purpose flour
1 cup whole wheat flour
1 teaspoon salt
1 teaspoon baking powder
½ teaspoon baking soda
1 tablespoon ground cinnamon
2 cups grated zucchini
1 pint blueberries

CHOOSE THIS!

Zucchini is a great source of folate, potassium, and vitamin A. At only about 25 calories each and the ability to quickly absorb flavors, zucchini make wonderful "fillers" to help you bulk up any dish with very little caloric or flavor impact.

1 Preheat oven to 350 degrees F. Spray two 9x9 inch baking dishes with nonstick cooking spray. You may also use silicone muffin, brownie, bar, or mini loaf pans.

2 In a large mixing bowl, whisk together egg white, apple sauce, vanilla extract, and sugar.

3 In a separate mixing bowl, combine flour, wheat flour, salt, baking powder, baking soda, and cinnamon.

4 Add the dry ingredients to the wet ingredients, stirring just until all is combined and a batter is formed.

5 Gently fold zucchini and blueberries into the batter and then divide equally between the two greased baking dishes.

6 Bake 35-40 minutes, until a toothpick inserted into the center of the bars comes out clean. Let cool 15 minutes before cutting each dish into 12 bars. Serve warm or at room temperature.

BOREDOM BUSTING BREAKFASTS

BANANA BREAD OATMEAL

"This easy and satisfying breakfast dish is cooked in only a few minutes in the microwave. Topping the oatmeal with sliced bananas and chopped pecans makes for a great presentation."

YOU WILL NEED

⅓ cup old-fashioned oats

¾ cup vanilla flavored soy milk

½ small banana, thinly sliced

1 tablespoon chopped pecans

1 teaspoon light agave nectar (may use honey)

1 Stir oats into the soy milk in a microwave-safe dish and microwave on high for 2-3 minutes, stirring halfway through. Oatmeal should be hot and bubbly.

2 Carefully remove from microwave and top with banana slices and chopped pecans.

3 Drizzle all with the agave nectar just before serving.

CHOOSE THIS!

Old-fashioned Oats, or "rolled" oats, had been almost entirely replaced by the popular quick-cooking oats, but finally they are back in style! The old-fashioned variety is less processed, leaving them higher in fiber and nutrients than quick-cooking oats. With only a few minutes of microwaving time either way, I find the difference in cooking time to be completely negligible.

CANADIAN BACON OMELET

"This heart-healthy omelet is made with egg whites, but you'll hardly miss the yolks. Sliced green onions are mixed right into the egg for even more flavor and a nice contrast to the Canadian bacon."

YOU WILL NEED

3 large egg whites

⅛ teaspoon salt

⅛ teaspoon pepper

⅛ teaspoon garlic powder

nonstick cooking spray

1 green onion, thinly sliced

2 full tablespoons shredded reduced-fat Cheddar cheese

3 slices Canadian bacon, diced

CHOOSE THIS!

Canadian Bacon has about ¼ the calories and ⅓ the saturated fat of regular bacon. Choosing delicious Canadian bacon, or even low-fat turkey bacon, is just one of those easy ways that you can change bad eating habits into good ones.

1 In a mixing bowl, whisk together egg whites, salt, pepper, and garlic powder until very frothy.

2 Spray a medium-sized nonstick skillet with nonstick cooking spray and place over medium-high heat.

3 Stir the sliced green onions into the frothy egg whites and then pour into the hot pan.

4 Cover pan and cook until the top of the whites are almost entirely set.

5 Sprinkle cheese over the entire surface of the egg whites and then arrange Canadian bacon only over half. Re-cover and cook an additional 15 seconds to melt cheese.

6 Gently fold the cheese-only side of the omelet over top of the side with the bacon. Serve immediately.

BOREDOM BUSTING BREAKFASTS

THE GIANT FRITTATA

"This giant frittata really earns its name! This is a perfect, fulfilling dish that allows you to feed the entire family a healthy breakfast with one single pan."

YOU WILL NEED

8 large egg whites

¼ cup grated Parmesan cheese

¼ teaspoon baking powder

⅛ teaspoon salt

⅛ teaspoon pepper

1 tablespoon olive oil

¼ cup diced yellow onion

½ cup diced red bell pepper

½ cup diced mushrooms

2 tablespoons fresh chopped parsley

CHOOSE THIS!

Parmesan Cheese is used in this frittata because its intense flavor allows you to use less cheese (which equals less calories and fat) than you would if using more mild choices like Cheddar or Monterey jack. The harder and more aged the Parmesan is, the more flavor it will pack, so grabbing a decent brand will definitely pay off.

1 Preheat broiler to high.

2 In a mixing bowl, beat egg whites until frothy. Stir in Parmesan cheese, baking powder, salt, and pepper.

3 Add olive oil to a large oven-safe skillet and place over medium-high heat.

4 Place onions in the hot skillet and cook until they begin to turn translucent. Add peppers and cook for 2 minutes before adding mushrooms. Cook 2 additional minutes.

5 Pour egg mixture over vegetables in skillet and cook about 4 minutes or until the top is beginning to set.

6 Place skillet into oven and broil for 3 minutes, just until the top begins to brown. Remove from oven, sprinkle with chopped parsley, and cut into 6 equal pieces to serve.

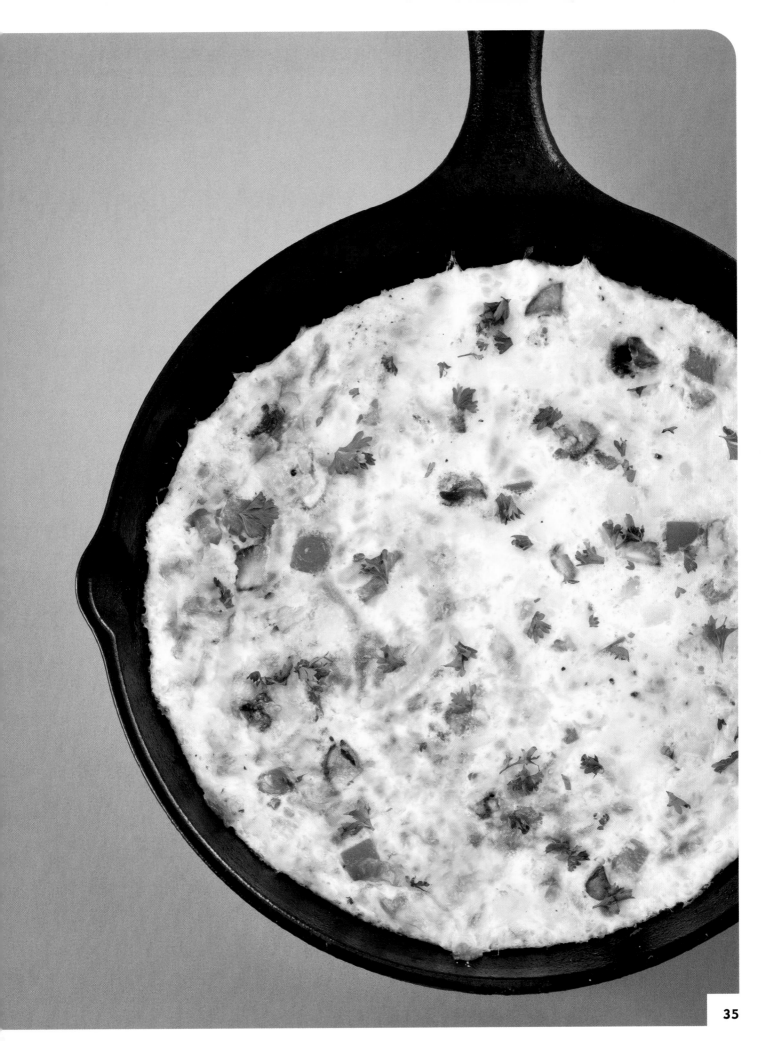

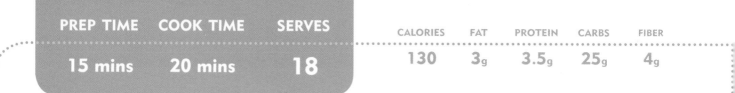

BRAN MUFFINS

"These deliciously spiced muffins are bursting with raisins, walnuts, and a healthy dose of whole grain goodness!"

YOU WILL NEED

1 cup Fiber One cereal
1 cup water
1 cup whole wheat flour
2 teaspoons baking powder
½ teaspoon salt
¼ teaspoon ground nutmeg
1 tablespoon ground cinnamon
½ cup old-fashioned oats
½ cup light brown sugar
1 large egg, beaten
½ cup unsweetened apple sauce
1 cup low-fat buttermilk
2 teaspoons vanilla extract
½ cup raisins
½ cup chopped walnuts

CHOOSE THIS!

Whole Grains, like those in the Fiber One cereal and whole wheat flour in this recipe, are much higher in vitamins, minerals, fiber, and antioxidants than refined or "white" grains. Studies have shown that eating more whole grains may help with weight management and reduce the risk of heart disease, cancer, and diabetes.

1 Preheat oven to 400 degrees F. Line muffin tins with 18 paper liners or simply use a silicone muffin or bar pan. For best results: spray paper liners with nonstick cooking spray.

2 In a large mixing bowl, place cereal in water and let stand while you continue preparing the other ingredients.

3 In another mixing bowl, combine flour, baking powder, salt, nutmeg, cinnamon, and oats.

4 Once the cereal has absorbed the water, add the brown sugar, egg, apple sauce, buttermilk, and vanilla extract, and stir to combine.

5 Add the dry ingredients to the wet ingredients, stirring just until combined. Gently fold raisins and walnuts into the batter.

6 Evenly divide batter into the prepared pans, making 18 muffins. Bake 20 minutes or until a toothpick inserted into the center of a muffin comes out mostly clean.

ITALIAN EGG SANDWICH

"This Italian Egg Sandwich substitutes a big slab of fresh, crisp tomato in place of the high-fat sausage or bacon you'd find in other egg sandwiches. Parmesan cheese adds a sharp cheese flavor with very few calories."

YOU WILL NEED

1 whole grain English muffin

1 thick slice tomato

1/8 teaspoon dry oregano

1 teaspoon olive oil

1 large egg

salt and pepper

1 tablespoon grated Parmesan cheese

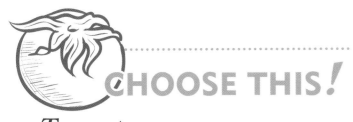

CHOOSE THIS!

Tomatoes are an excellent source of vitamins A, C, and K, but it's this mostly-savory fruit's lycopene content that truly sets it apart. Lycopene may reduce the risk for certain cancers and can even help maintain healthy blood pressure and strong bones. Eating tomatoes with a small amount of fat, like the egg yolk and olive oil in this recipe, can actually help the body to absorb that precious lycopene.

1 Toast or lightly grill English muffin, and place the thick slice of tomato onto the bottom half. Sprinkle oregano over tomato slice.

2 Add olive oil to a small nonstick skillet and place over medium-high heat.

3 Crack egg into the hot skillet and sprinkle with a small amount of salt and pepper. Note: break yolk if you don't like it runny!

4 Add a teaspoon or two of water to the pan, cover, and cook until the top of the egg is set.

5 Sprinkle cheese over the egg, re-cover, and cook just until cheese begins to melt.

6 Transfer the cooked egg to the top of the tomato and cover with the other half of the English muffin to complete the sandwich.

BOREDOM BUSTING BREAKFASTS

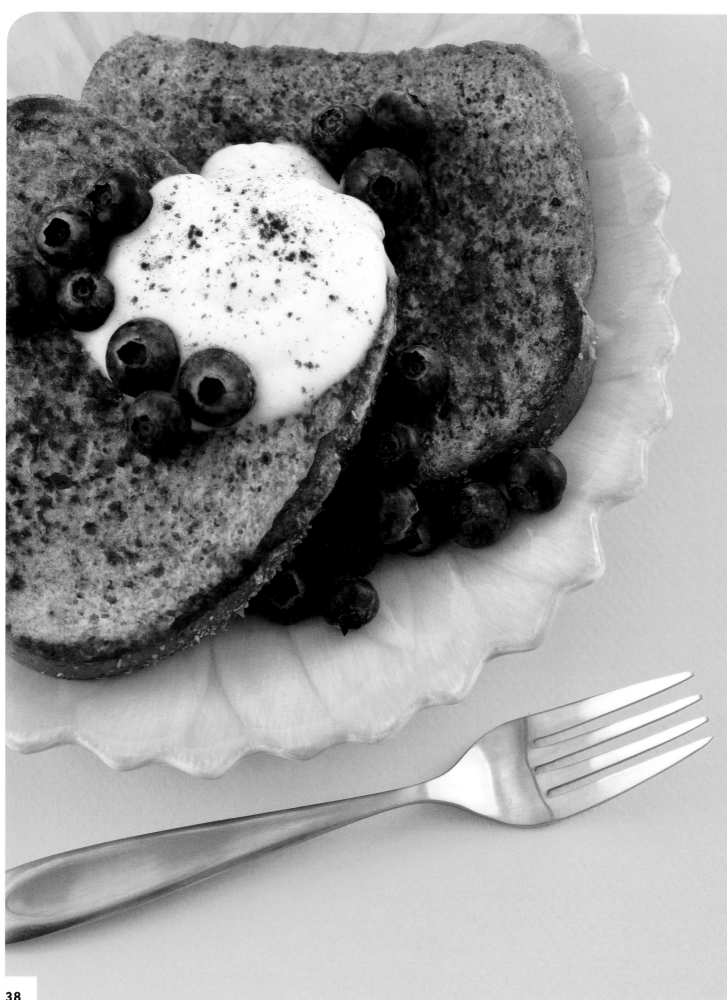

BETTER FOR YOU FRENCH TOAST

"I've always found that using whole eggs, including the saturated fat-filled yolk, is rather unnecessary when preparing French toast! My recipe uses only the whites and then tops the finished toast with yogurt and fruit for a healthy breakfast with a great presentation."

YOU WILL NEED

3 large egg whites

1 tablespoon water

½ teaspoon vanilla extract

1 teaspoon ground cinnamon

nonstick cooking spray

4 slices whole wheat bread

½ cup nonfat plain yogurt

2 tablespoons light agave nectar (may use honey)

1 cup blueberries (or mixed berries)

CHOOSE THIS!

Egg Whites are pure protein without the calories, fat, or cholesterol of whole eggs. In most recipes, including baked goods, 2 egg whites can easily substitute 1 whole egg with very little impact on the final dish.

1 In a mixing bowl, beat together egg whites, water, vanilla extract, and cinnamon.

2 Spray a large skillet or griddle with nonstick cooking spray and place over medium heat.

3 Dip one slice of bread at a time into the egg mixture, coating both sides. Add the coated bread to the pan, cooking 2 at a time or all 4 if they will fit.

4 Cook until the bread is golden brown on the bottom and then flip to cook the other side.

5 Meanwhile, combine yogurt and agave nectar to make a yogurt topping.

6 Serve 2 slices of French toast on each plate, topped with ½ of the yogurt topping and ½ of the blueberries.

BOREDOM BUSTING BREAKFASTS

CARROT CAKE MUFFINS

"These spiced breakfast muffins with carrots mixed right into the batter are just like carrot cake without the high-calorie frosting. It's still breakfast so frosting can definitely wait!"

YOU WILL NEED

1 ¾ cups all-purpose flour

¾ cup light brown sugar

2 teaspoons baking powder

1 teaspoon baking soda

½ teaspoon ground nutmeg

¼ teaspoon ground ginger

1 teaspoon ground cinnamon

½ teaspoon salt

¾ cup nonfat plain yogurt

4 tablespoons butter, melted

1 teaspoon vanilla extract

1 large egg

¼ cup fat-free milk

1 ¾ cups shredded carrots

1 Preheat oven to 375 degrees F. Line muffin tins with 12 paper liners, or simply use a silicone muffin or bar pan.

2 In a mixing bowl, combine flour, brown sugar, baking powder, baking soda, nutmeg, ginger, cinnamon, and salt.

3 In a separate mixing bowl, whisk together yogurt, melted butter, vanilla extract, egg, and milk.

4 Add the dry ingredients to the wet ingredients, stirring just until combined and a batter is formed. Fold carrots into the batter.

5 Evenly divide batter into the prepared pans, making 12 muffins. Bake 18-20 minutes or until a toothpick inserted into the center of a muffin comes out mostly clean. Let cool 10 minutes before serving warm or at room temperature.

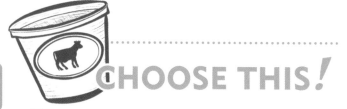

CHOOSE THIS!

Yogurt, as most people know, is a good source of protein and calcium. It also contains beneficial probiotics that can aid in digestion and inhibit harmful bacteria from growing in your body, which boosts immunity.

FULLY LOADED GRANOLA

"Granola is one of those long recognized "health foods" because of its nourishing and satisfying whole grains, fruits, nuts, and seeds. However, granola's one downfall has often been its high fat and calorie content due to added oil. My recipe gets nice and crisp without ANY added oil."

YOU WILL NEED

3 ½ cups old-fashioned oats

1 cup shredded coconut

¾ cup sliced almonds

¼ cup ground flax seeds

2 teaspoons ground cinnamon

½ cup light brown sugar

½ cup light agave nectar (may use honey)

¼ cup apple sauce

½ teaspoon salt

2 teaspoons almond extract

½ cup dried cherries

CHOOSE THIS!

Apple Sauce is used in this recipe to creatively replace the oil that would traditionally be used. This tried and true trick also works well in most baking recipes, especially those for muffins.

1 Preheat oven to 325 degrees F.

2 In a large mixing bowl, combine oats, coconut, almonds, flax seeds, and cinnamon.

3 Place brown sugar, agave nectar, apple sauce, and salt in a sauce pan over medium heat and bring to a simmer. Simmer for 1 minute. Remove from heat and stir in almond extract.

4 Pour the hot liquid mixture over the dry ingredients in the mixing bowl and toss all to combine.

5 Spread mixture onto a large sheet pan and bake 25 minutes, stirring occasionally.

6 Remove from oven and let cool in pan until it reaches room temperature. Use a metal spatula to release from pan. Release from pan and toss with the dried cherries to finish. Store in an airtight container.

BOREDOM BUSTING BREAKFASTS

SAVORY QUICHE CUPS

"Quiche has a reputation for being high in calories and fat (and for good reason), but I've carefully crafted these mini versions down to only 175 calories each!"

YOU WILL NEED

nonstick cooking spray

1 sheet frozen puffed pastry (such as Pillsbury), thawed

4 large eggs

1 cup fat-free half and half

¼ cup shredded Parmesan cheese

½ cup shredded part-skim mozzarella cheese

1 tomato, diced

¼ cup fresh spinach leaves, chopped

¼ teaspoon salt

⅛ teaspoon pepper

CHOOSE THIS!

Fat-Free Dairy, such as the fat-free half and half used in this recipe, can save you a ton of calories over their full-fat alternatives while still giving you most of the creaminess you are looking for. A typical quiche recipe would use heavy cream that has 45 grams of fat per cup!

1 Preheat oven to 350 degrees F. Spray a 12 cup muffin tin with nonstick cooking spray.

2 Unfold puffed pastry and cut into 12 equal squares. Press 1 square into each cup of a muffin tin and prick the bottom a few times with a fork.

3 In a mixing bowl, beat the eggs and half and half until combined. Stir in Parmesan cheese, mozzarella cheese, diced tomato, chopped spinach, salt, and pepper.

4 Divide the egg mixture evenly between the 12 pastry-lined muffin cups.

5 Bake 25 minutes, or until a toothpick inserted into the center of a quiche cup comes out mostly clean. Serve warm or chilled.

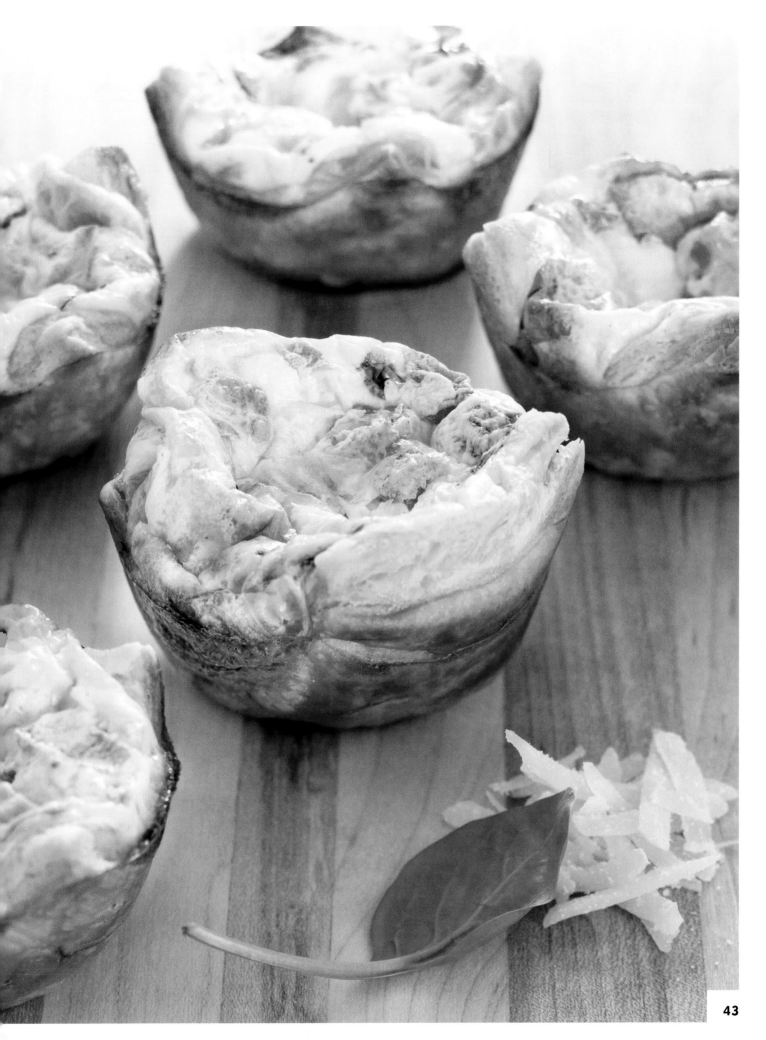

PUMPKIN PATCH PANCAKES

"As I'm sure you can see from other recipes in this book, I absolutely love canned pumpkin! It's not only nutritious, but it also couldn't be any easier to use. In this recipe, it gives these pancakes a smooth and creamy consistency without an abundance of added oil or butter."

YOU WILL NEED

1 cup whole wheat flour

2 teaspoons baking powder

1 teaspoon baking soda

½ teaspoon pumpkin pie spice

1 tablespoon light agave nectar (may use honey)

1 ½ cups soy milk (may use almond or skim milk)

⅓ cup canned pumpkin

1 tablespoon olive oil

nonstick cooking spray

CHOOSE THIS!

Pumpkin is extremely high in anti-oxidants and beta-carotene, which can help regenerate cells in the body. This effect makes it a great "age reversing" food. Its smooth consistency helps keep these pancakes moist with very little added oil.

1 In a mixing bowl, combine the flour, baking powder, baking soda, and pumpkin pie spice, stirring well.

2 Add the agave nectar, soy milk, canned pumpkin, and olive oil, and mix all until just combined.

3 Spray a large skillet or griddle with nonstick cooking spray and place over medium heat.

4 Pour ¼ cup of batter into the skillet for each pancake, adding as many as will fit.

5 Cook until bubbles begin to form on the surface, about 2 minutes, before flipping and cooking until golden brown, about 2 additional minutes. Repeat until all batter is exhausted.

6 Serve with sugar-free maple syrup or drizzle with additional agave nectar and top with fresh fruit.

PREP TIME	COOK TIME	SERVES		CALORIES	FAT	PROTEIN	CARBS	FIBER
15 mins	10 mins	1		295	13g	18g	29g	6g

WHOLE WHEAT BREAKFAST BURRITOS

"This burrito has everything you need for a well balanced breakfast and then some! Feel free to double, triple, or quadruple the recipe to feed the whole family."

YOU WILL NEED

1 large egg

1 large egg white

3 drops hot sauce

⅛ teaspoon salt

⅛ teaspoon pepper

nonstick cooking spray

1 green onion, thinly sliced

¼ cup diced red bell pepper

¼ cup diced tomatoes

2 tablespoons shredded pepper-jack cheese

1 tablespoon fresh chopped cilantro

1 whole wheat tortilla

1 In a mixing bowl, whisk together egg, egg white, hot sauce, salt, and pepper until frothy.

2 Spray a nonstick skillet with nonstick cooking spray and place over medium-high heat.

3 Add sliced green onion and diced bell pepper to the hot pan and cook until soft, about 2-3 minutes.

4 Add the beaten eggs and diced tomatoes to the skillet and stir together to scramble as the eggs set.

5 Once eggs are completely scrambled, top with the cheese and cilantro. Cover pan and remove from heat. Let sit 30 seconds for the cheese to melt.

6 Wrap tortilla in two sheets of paper towels and microwave 20-30 seconds to warm. Transfer the finished egg mixture to the warmed tortilla and roll up to serve.

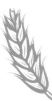

CHOOSE THIS!

Whole Grains like those in the whole wheat tortilla in this recipe are much higher in vitamins, minerals, fiber, and antioxidants than refined or "white" grains. Studies have shown that eating more whole grains may help with weight management and reduce the risk of heart disease, cancer, and diabetes.

BOREDOM BUSTING BREAKFASTS

ALL WRAPPED UP IN SANDWICHES

"Making a good, nutritious sandwich or wrap is one of my favorite ways to experiment in the kitchen. The possibilities are limitless."

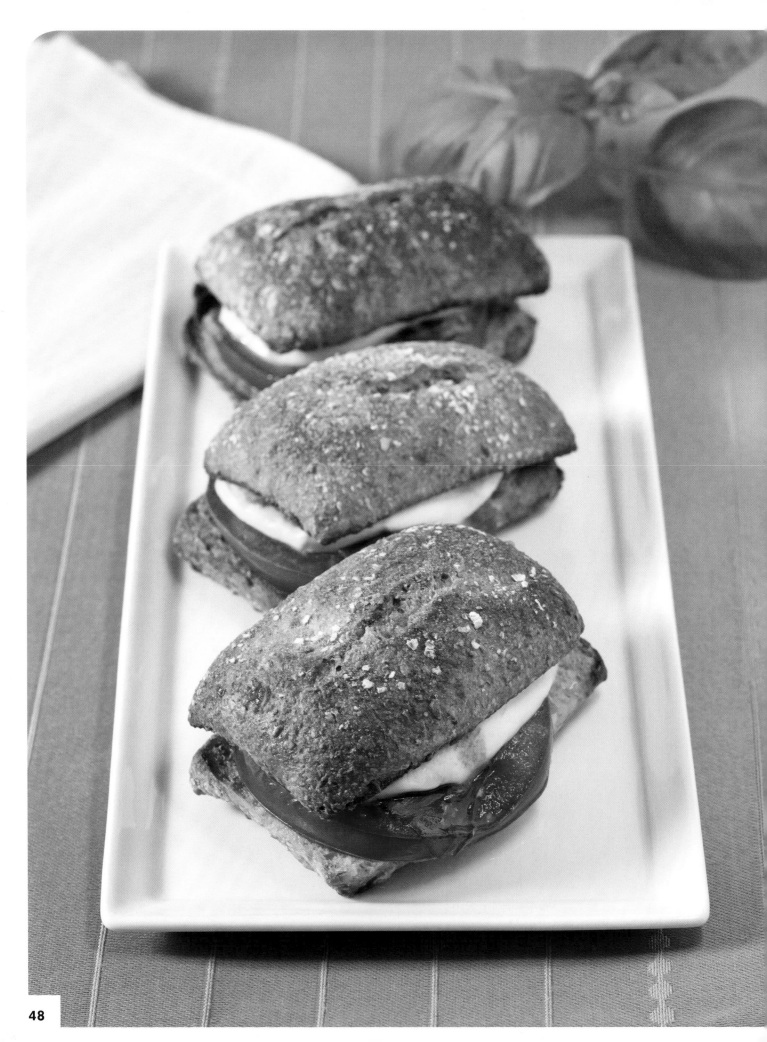

CAPRESE SANDWICHES

"This is a warmed version of a classic tomato and mozzarella salad, which is served between a healthy and hearty whole wheat roll that has been seasoned and broiled like garlic bread. You can think of it as an Italian grilled cheese sandwich!"

YOU WILL NEED

6 whole wheat rolls

2 tablespoons olive oil

2 teaspoons minced garlic

⅛ teaspoon salt

⅛ teaspoon pepper

1 large tomato, cut into 6 slices

12 fresh basil leaves

8 ounces fresh mozzarella, cut into 6 slices

2 tablespoons balsamic vinegar

2 teaspoons honey

CHOOSE THIS!

Basil, especially the fresh basil used in this recipe, is a very good source of vitamin A, which may help prevent free radicals from oxidizing cholesterol in your blood, keeping the cholesterol from building up in your blood vessels.

1 Preheat broiler to high. Separate rolls and place all 12 halves onto a sheet pan.

2 Combine olive oil, garlic, salt, and pepper and then lightly spread mixture onto the insides of all 12 halves of bread.

3 Top the bottom halves of the rolls with a slice of tomato, 2 basil leaves, and a slice of mozzarella cheese, in that order.

4 Position sheet pan about 6 inches from the broiler and cook 3-4 minutes, just until cheese is bubbling and buns are beginning to brown.

5 Meanwhile, combine vinegar and honey. Remove the sheet pan from the oven and lightly drizzle vinegar mixture over the melted mozzarella cheese.

6 Place each top bun into place to complete the sandwiches. Serve immediately.

ALL WRAPPED UP IN SANDWICHES

SALMON BURGERS

"These satisfying salmon burgers are made from whole chunks of fresh salmon and are topped with a creamy cilantro and lemon sauce in place of the typical (and high-fat) tartar sauce."

YOU WILL NEED

½ cup nonfat plain Greek yogurt

¼ cup fresh cilantro, chopped

3 tablespoons lemon juice

1 pound raw salmon, finely chopped

3 tablespoons whole wheat breadcrumbs

⅓ cup finely diced red bell pepper

5 green onions, thinly sliced

1 tablespoon prepared horseradish

1 large egg white

¼ teaspoon salt

⅛ teaspoon pepper

nonstick cooking spray

6 whole wheat buns, toasted

2 tomatoes, thinly sliced

CHOOSE THIS!

Salmon is a great source of essential omega-3 fatty acids, which are anti-inflammatory and play many important roles inside our bodies. These fatty acids are in fact essential, but our bodies do not create them on their own, so they must be present somewhere in our diet.

1 In a small mixing bowl, combine yogurt, ½ of the cilantro, and lemon juice to make a cilantro sauce. Season with salt and pepper to taste and refrigerate until serving.

2 In a large mixing bowl, thoroughly combine salmon, breadcrumbs, red bell pepper, green onions, horseradish, egg white, salt, pepper, and remaining cilantro.

3 Spray a large nonstick skillet with nonstick cooking spray and place over medium heat.

4 Form the salmon mixture into 6 equal patties and place in the hot pan, cooking for 4-5 minutes on each side, or until browned on the outside and cooked throughout.

5 Place cooked salmon burgers on toasted buns and top with sliced tomato and cilantro sauce before serving.

BLACK BEAN BURRITOS

"These vegetarian burritos are absolutely filled to the brim with whole grain brown rice and smothered in Mexican seasoned black beans. Like all great burritos, there is definitely cheese involved!"

YOU WILL NEED

2 tablespoons olive oil

¼ cup diced red onion

2 cloves garlic, minced

½ teaspoon cumin

1 tablespoon canned diced jalapeños

1 (14.5-ounce) can diced tomatoes

1 (15-ounce) can black beans, drained and rinsed

½ cup fresh cilantro, chopped

salt and pepper

4 whole wheat tortillas

2 cups cooked brown rice

1 ½ cups shredded reduced-fat Cheddar-jack cheese

1 Place oil in a large skillet over medium heat. Once hot, add onions and sauté until onions are translucent.

2 Add garlic and cumin to the pan and cook an additional 1 minute before adding jalapeños, tomatoes (with liquid), and black beans.

3 Let mixture cook until the liquid from the tomatoes begins to thicken, about 8-10 minutes. Remove from heat and stir in cilantro and salt and pepper to taste.

4 Assemble burritos by filling each whole wheat tortilla with ¼ of the brown rice and a good amount of the hot bean mixture. Top bean mixture with ¼ of the cheese and then fold in sides of the tortilla to roll up and serve.

CHOOSE THIS!

Black Beans, like most beans and legumes, are a very good source of fiber. Fiber can not only help aid in digestion and lower cholesterol but can also prevent blood sugar levels from rising too rapidly after meals. It is this effect that keeps you feeling full and satisfied longer, which keeps you from overeating.

ALL WRAPPED UP IN SANDWICHES

PREP TIME	COOK TIME	SERVES		CALORIES	FAT	PROTEIN	CARBS	FIBER
20 mins	12 mins	4		297	12g	27.5g	20g	3.5g

SPINACH AND FETA STUFFED TURKEY BURGERS

"It's no secret that turkey burgers have a tendency to dry out, but stuffing them with spinach is a pretty good way to solve that problem. As the moisture cooks out of the spinach, it has nowhere else to go but into the burgers, keeping them nice and juicy."

YOU WILL NEED

1 pound lean ground turkey

2 tablespoons finely minced yellow onion

½ teaspoon dried oregano

⅛ teaspoon garlic powder

¼ teaspoon salt

¼ teaspoon pepper

1 cup frozen chopped spinach, thawed and drained

⅓ cup crumbled feta cheese

1 teaspoon minced garlic

4 whole wheat buns

CHOOSE THIS!

Spinach is rich in vitamins, minerals, and antioxidants. It also contains choline and inositol, which can prevent hardening of the arteries. When using frozen spinach, I prefer to purchase the bags of chopped spinach as they thaw faster because they are not frozen into one single brick like the small boxes are.

1 In a mixing bowl, combine ground turkey, yellow onion, oregano, garlic powder, salt, and pepper, folding together with your hands.

2 Form ground turkey mixture into 8 thin patties.

3 In a separate mixing bowl, fold together spinach, feta cheese, and minced garlic to create the burger filling.

4 Place a heaping spoonful of the filling onto the center of 4 of the thin burger patties. Place the other 4 thin patties over top of the filling topped patties and press down around the edges, crimping to seal the filling inside. You should now have 4 stuffed burger patties.

5 Oil and preheat a grill, indoor grill, or grill pan to high. Grill burgers for about 6 minutes on each side, or until cutting into one reveals no pink. Serve on whole wheat buns with your favorite burger fixings.

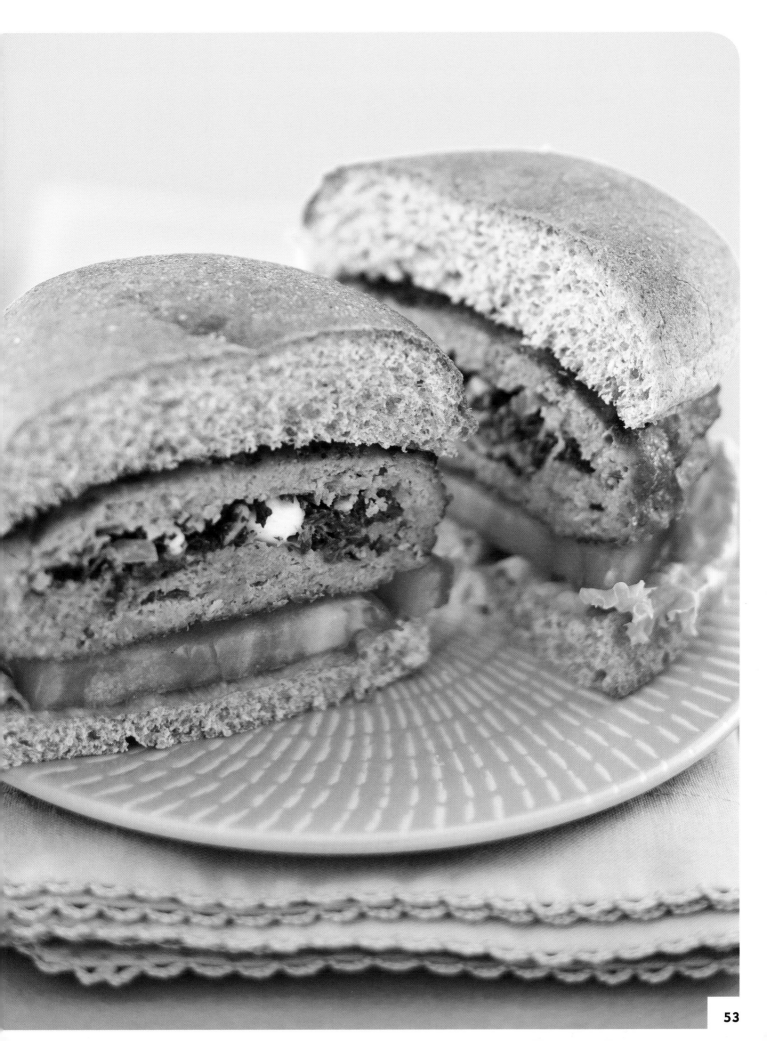

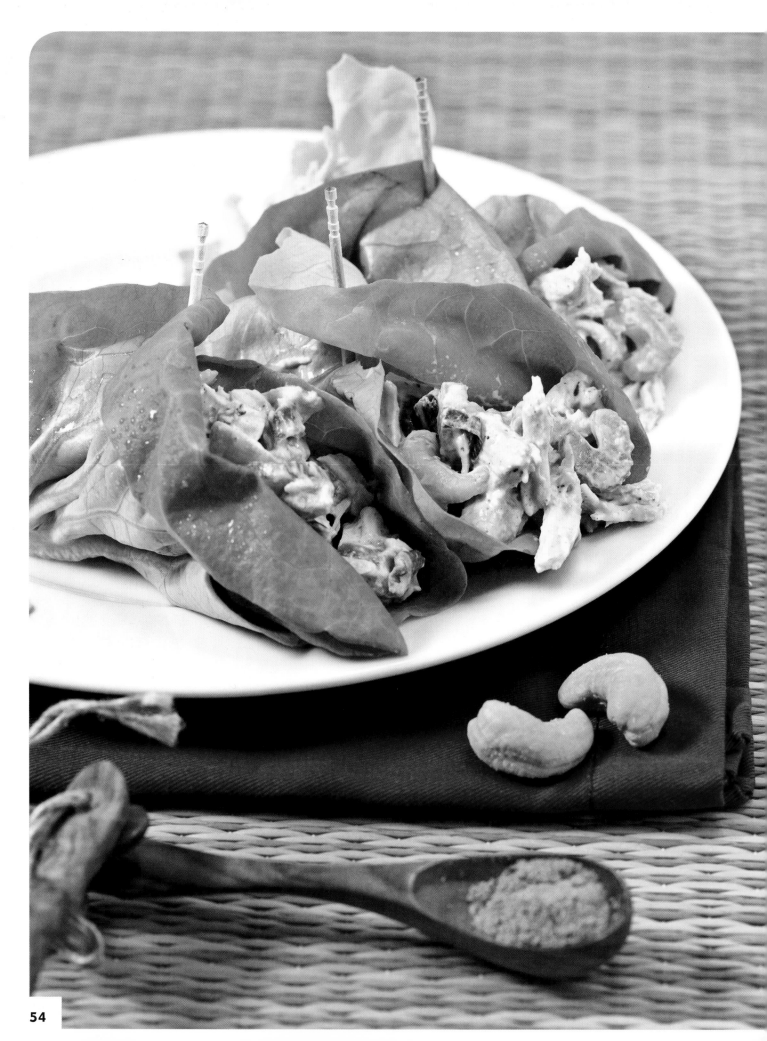

CURRY CHICKEN LETTUCE WRAPS

"These handy lettuce wraps are filled with a delicious and creamy curry chicken salad. Cashews add a nice, sweet crunch that offsets the stronger, spicier flavors of the curry powder."

YOU WILL NEED

2 cups shredded store-bought rotisserie chicken, skin removed

½ cup nonfat plain Greek yogurt

1 cup sliced celery

3 green onions, sliced

½ cup chopped cashews

1 ¼ teaspoons curry powder

¼ teaspoon salt

⅛ teaspoon pepper

8 large butter lettuce leaves, rinsed

1 In a large mixing bowl, combine shredded chicken, yogurt, celery, onions, cashews, curry powder, salt, and pepper to create a Curry Chicken Salad.

2 Lay out lettuce leaves and scoop an equal amount of the chicken salad into the center of each leaf.

3 Starting at one end, roll the stuffed lettuce leaves into a wrap, placing seam-side down to hold together. Serve chilled.

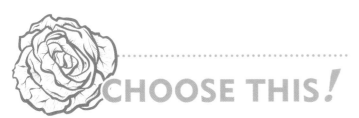

CHOOSE THIS!

Lettuce makes a wonderful and low-carbohydrate substitution for white or even whole wheat wraps or bread. While I do appreciate good whole grain bread for its great fiber content, skipping the bread in these wraps saves at least 100 calories.

ALL WRAPPED UP IN SANDWICHES

EGG SALAD PITA POCKETS

"These Egg Salad Pita Pockets are stuffed with an egg salad that is made with extra egg whites and creamy Greek yogurt for extra protein with less calories and cholesterol than your typical egg salad."

YOU WILL NEED

4 hardboiled eggs, 2 yolks removed

¼ cup diced celery

2 tablespoons nonfat plain Greek yogurt (may use regular yogurt)

2 teaspoons Dijon mustard

1 teaspoon dried dill

⅛ teaspoon salt

⅛ teaspoon pepper

2 pieces whole wheat pita bread

½ cup fresh spinach leaves

1 Finely dice the hardboiled egg whites and whole eggs and then add to a mixing bowl.

2 Add the celery, yogurt, mustard, dill, salt, and pepper to the bowl and fold together until all is combined.

3 Cut each piece of pita bread in half and then open each half into a pocket.

4 Stuff each pita pocket with an equal amount of spinach leaves and egg salad before serving. Makes 2 servings of 2 pockets each.

CHOOSE THIS!

Egg Whites of two eggs are used in this recipe to bulk this salad up without using 4 whole eggs. This reduces the overall number of calories and the amount of cholesterol in this recipe by a significant amount. For a completely different salad with a similar texture but even fewer calories and no cholesterol, substitute the eggs with about 1 cup of diced tofu.

SUNFLOWER TURKEY WRAPS

"These simple sandwich wraps are smothered in fat-free cream cheese rather than high-cholesterol mayonnaise. Topping with dried cranberries and sunflower seeds makes an otherwise ordinary wrap into something extraordinary!"

YOU WILL NEED

1 whole wheat flour tortilla

2 tablespoons fat-free cream cheese

1 tablespoon dried cranberries

1 tablespoon sunflower seeds, shelled

¼ pound deli sliced turkey breast

¼ cup fresh spinach leaves

2 tablespoons shredded carrots

1 Lay the tortilla flat and cover the entire surface with the fat-free cream cheese.

2 Top cream cheese with the dried cranberries and sunflower seeds, and press them down lightly to stick.

3 Pile the turkey breast, spinach leaves, and shredded carrots down the center of the tortilla.

4 Starting at one end, roll the stuffed tortilla into a wrap, allowing the cream cheese to seal it together. Slice in half and serve.

CHOOSE THIS!

Sunflower Seeds are an excellent source of vitamin E, magnesium, and selenium. Vitamin E travels through the body neutralizing free radicals that could otherwise damage cells and promote cardiovascular disease. Magnesium like that found in sunflower seeds helps in producing energy in the body, making it vital for an active lifestyle!

ALL WRAPPED UP IN SANDWICHES

PREP TIME	COOK TIME	SERVES		CALORIES	FAT	PROTEIN	CARBS	FIBER
15 mins	5 mins	6		230	15g	6.5g	10.5g	4g

VERY VEGGIE BAGUETTE SANDWICHES

"With fresh veggies, feta cheese, and chopped walnuts piled high on a crusty whole grain baguette slathered with stone ground mustard, this sandwich is a delicious and unique combination of fresh flavors."

YOU WILL NEED

1 whole grain baguette

6 tablespoons stone ground mustard

1 cup fresh arugula (may use fresh baby spinach)

1 avocado, thinly sliced

2 Roma tomatoes, thinly sliced

1 cucumber, peeled and thinly sliced

4 ounces crumbled feta cheese

½ cup chopped walnuts

1 Preheat oven to 350 degrees F. Slice baguette in half lengthwise, separating into two long pieces.

2 Place directly on oven rack and bake 5 minutes, just until lightly toasted.

3 Carefully remove baguette halves from oven and spread both with mustard.

4 Layer arugula, avocado, tomatoes, cucumber, feta cheese, and walnuts equally over the bottom half of the baguette.

5 Cover bottom of baguette with the top half and cut into 6 equal sandwiches before serving.

CHOOSE THIS!

Walnuts are an excellent source of omega-3 essential fatty acids, which are a special type of protective fat that the body cannot make on its own. Not just that, but Walnuts also offer many other health benefits including cardiovascular protection, the promotion of better cognitive function, and even anti-inflammatory benefits.

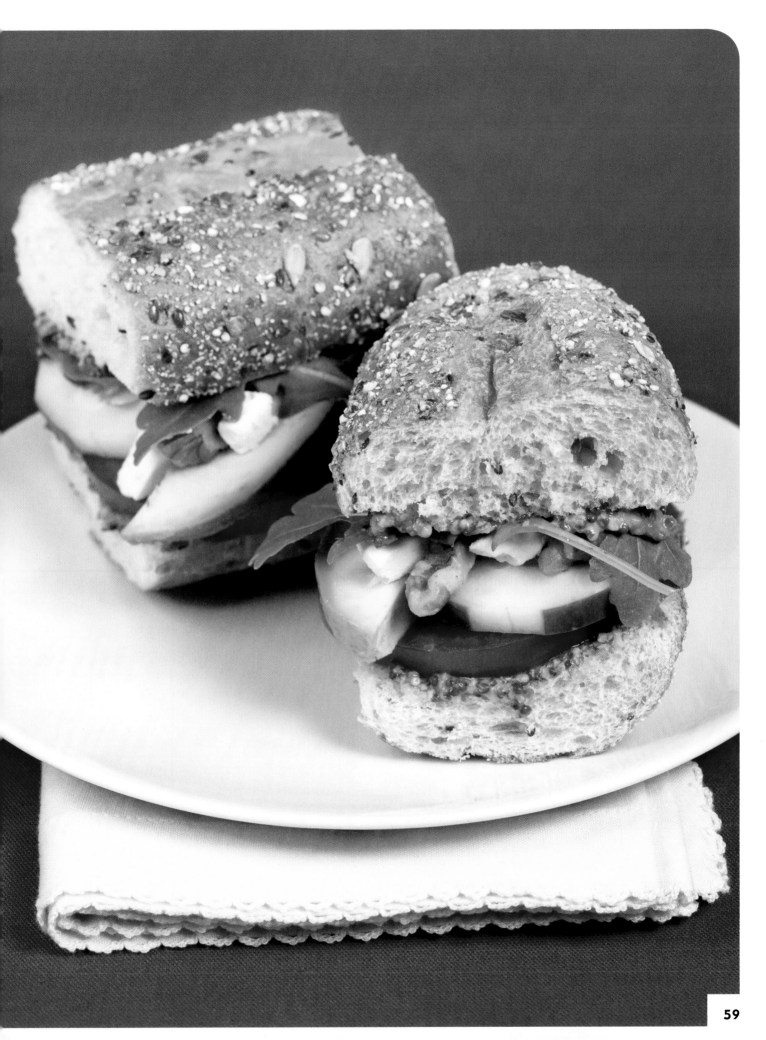

ROASTED RED PEPPER AND HUMMUS WRAPS

"These wraps begin with a spreading of rich and creamy hummus and are then topped with smoky and sweet roasted red peppers. Toasted pine nuts, julienned cucumber, shredded carrots, and romaine lettuce round these wraps out and lend them a very satisfying crunch."

YOU WILL NEED

½ cup pine nuts

4 whole wheat tortillas

½ cup hummus

1 jarred roasted red pepper, thinly sliced

1 cucumber, julienned

1 cup shredded carrots

1 ½ cups chopped romaine lettuce

CHOOSE THIS!

Hummus is made from puréed garbanzo beans (also known as chickpeas). Garbanzo beans, like most beans and legumes, are a great source of cholesterol-lowering and blood sugar stabilizing fiber. This makes hummus a great substitute for creamy condiments like mayonnaise, which are pretty void of important nutrients.

1 Preheat oven to 400 degrees F. Place pine nuts on a sheet pan and bake for 5-6 minutes, tossing halfway through. Cook just until the pine nuts are golden brown (toasted) and very fragrant.

2 Lay out whole wheat tortillas and spread the entire surface of each with 2 tablespoons of the hummus.

3 Sprinkle pine nuts down one side of each tortilla and then top with an equal amount of all remaining ingredients, keeping everything to that same side.

4 Roll the filled tortillas up into wraps and slice in half to serve.

STUFFED "PIZZA" BURGERS

"These burgers made with lean ground beef are literally stuffed with pizza sauce and mozzarella cheese for a taste that kids are sure to love. I like them with diced green bell pepper for more of that "supreme" pizza taste, but you can leave that out if serving to picky kids."

YOU WILL NEED

1 pound extra-lean ground beef

2 tablespoons grated Parmesan cheese

2 teaspoons minced garlic

½ teaspoon Italian seasoning

¼ teaspoon salt

¼ teaspoon pepper

⅓ cup shredded mozzarella cheese

2 tablespoons finely diced green bell pepper

¼ teaspoon dried oregano

¼ cup jarred pizza sauce

4 whole wheat buns

CHOOSE THIS!

Lean Beef can be a very healthy source of protein with a very high amount of iron, magnesium, and zinc. Ground round is usually the leanest type of ground beef, followed by ground sirloin. Both can contain far less fat than regular ground turkey or chicken!

1 In a mixing bowl, combine ground beef, Parmesan cheese, garlic, Italian seasoning, salt, and pepper, folding together with your hands.

2 Form ground beef mixture into 8 thin patties.

3 In a separate mixing bowl, fold together mozzarella cheese, bell pepper, and dried oregano to create the burger filling.

4 Spread a spoonful of the pizza sauce onto the center of 4 of the thin burger patties and then top with a heaping spoonful of the filling. Place the other 4 thin patties over top of the filling topped patties and press down around the edges, crimping to seal the filling inside. You should now have 4 stuffed burger patties.

5 Oil and preheat a grill, indoor grill, or grill pan to high. Grill burgers for 5-6 minutes on each side for medium-well doneness. Serve on whole wheat buns with your favorite burger fixings.

ALL WRAPPED UP IN SANDWICHES

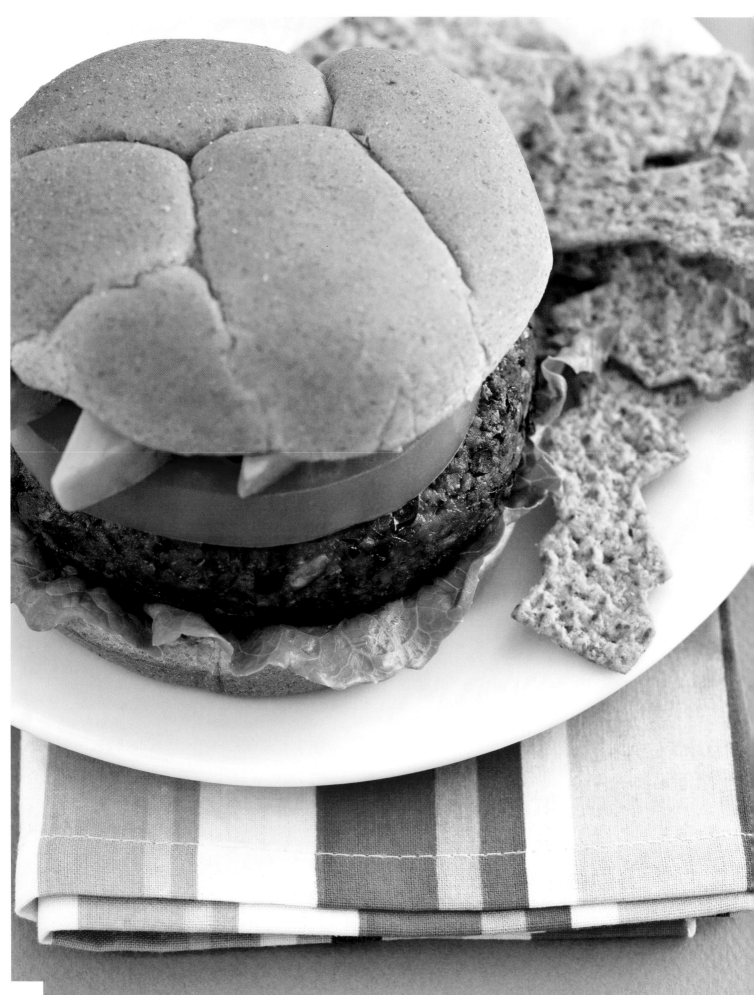

PREP TIME	COOK TIME	SERVES		CALORIES	FAT	PROTEIN	CARBS	FIBER
25 mins	10 mins	4		390	13.5g	17g	60g	15.5g

SPICY BLACK BEAN BURGERS

"These vegetarian burgers are bursting with black beans and made all the more delicious (and spicy) by having pepper-jack cheese mixed throughout the burgers themselves."

YOU WILL NEED

1 (15-ounce) can black beans, drained and rinsed
½ cup whole wheat breadcrumbs
1 large egg white
2 cloves garlic, minced
¼ cup diced red onion
½ cup fresh cilantro
1 teaspoon chili powder
½ teaspoon cumin
¼ teaspoon salt
⅛ teaspoon pepper
½ cup shredded pepper-jack cheese
nonstick cooking spray
4 whole wheat buns, toasted
1 avocado, peeled and sliced

CHOOSE THIS!

Black Beans, like most beans and legumes, are a very good source of fiber. Fiber can not only help aid in digestion and lower cholesterol but can also prevent blood sugar levels from rising too rapidly after meals.

1 In the bowl of a food processor, combine the black beans, breadcrumbs, egg white, garlic, red onion, cilantro, chili powder, cumin, salt, and pepper. Pulse until mixture is well combined and beans are finely chopped but not entirely smooth.

2 Fold pepper-jack cheese into the blended bean mixture.

3 Spray a large nonstick skillet with non-stick cooking spray and place over medium heat.

4 Form the bean and cheese mixture into 4 equal patties and place in the hot pan, cooking for 3-4 minutes on each side, or until hot throughout.

5 Place cooked black bean burgers on toasted buns and top with sliced avocado before serving.

ALL WRAPPED UP IN SANDWICHES

GRILLED CHICKEN GYROS

"These wrapped Greek sandwiches are filled with oregano-marinated chicken and topped with tzatziki, a creamy cucumber and dill sauce."

YOU WILL NEED

1 pound boneless, skinless chicken breasts

1 tablespoon olive oil

1 teaspoon dried oregano

¼ teaspoon salt

⅛ teaspoon pepper

⅛ teaspoon garlic powder

1 cucumber, peeled

½ cup nonfat plain Greek yogurt

1 tablespoon lemon juice

2 teaspoons fresh chopped dill

1 teaspoon minced garlic

4 multi-grain flatbreads or pitas

1 cup cherry tomatoes, quartered

¼ cup diced red onion

¼ cup crumbled feta cheese

CHOOSE THIS!

Greek Yogurt is becoming more and more popular in America, and it is for a good reason! Not only is Greek yogurt far thicker than regular yogurt, but it also has a higher concentration of protein and probiotics.

1 Slice chicken breasts into ½ inch strips and place in a plastic storage bag or container. Add olive oil, oregano, salt, pepper, and garlic powder to the bag, seal, and shake to fully coat chicken. Refrigerate for at least 30 minutes to marinate.

2 Begin preparing the Greek tzatziki sauce by finely dicing ½ of the cucumber. For best results, cut the seeds and clear membrane out of the cucumber and discard before dicing. Chop the other ½ of the cucumber into ½ inch cubes and set aside for topping the gyro.

3 Place the finely diced cucumber in a mixing bowl and add yogurt, lemon juice, dill, and garlic, stirring to combine all. Add salt to taste and then refrigerate until ready to serve gyros.

4 Preheat a grill, an indoor grill, or grill pan to high. Remove chicken from marinade and grill 7-8 minutes, turning once, until cutting into a strip reveals no pink.

5 Assemble the gyros by placing an equal amount of the chicken down the center of each of the 4 flatbreads. Top with an equal amount of the cubed cucumber, tomatoes, red onion, and feta cheese.

6 Spoon tzatziki sauce over gyros and fold up to serve.

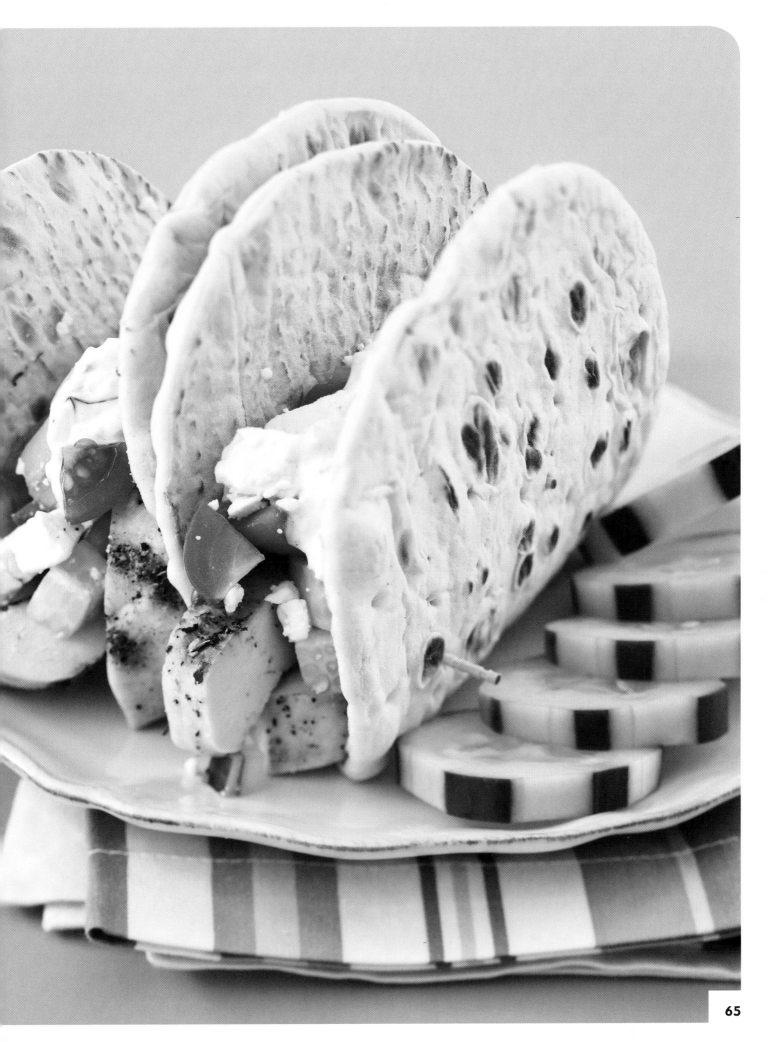

LETTUCE EAT SALAD

· ·

"These are some of my favorite recipes for unique and nutritious green salads and picnic salads, which make great side dishes."

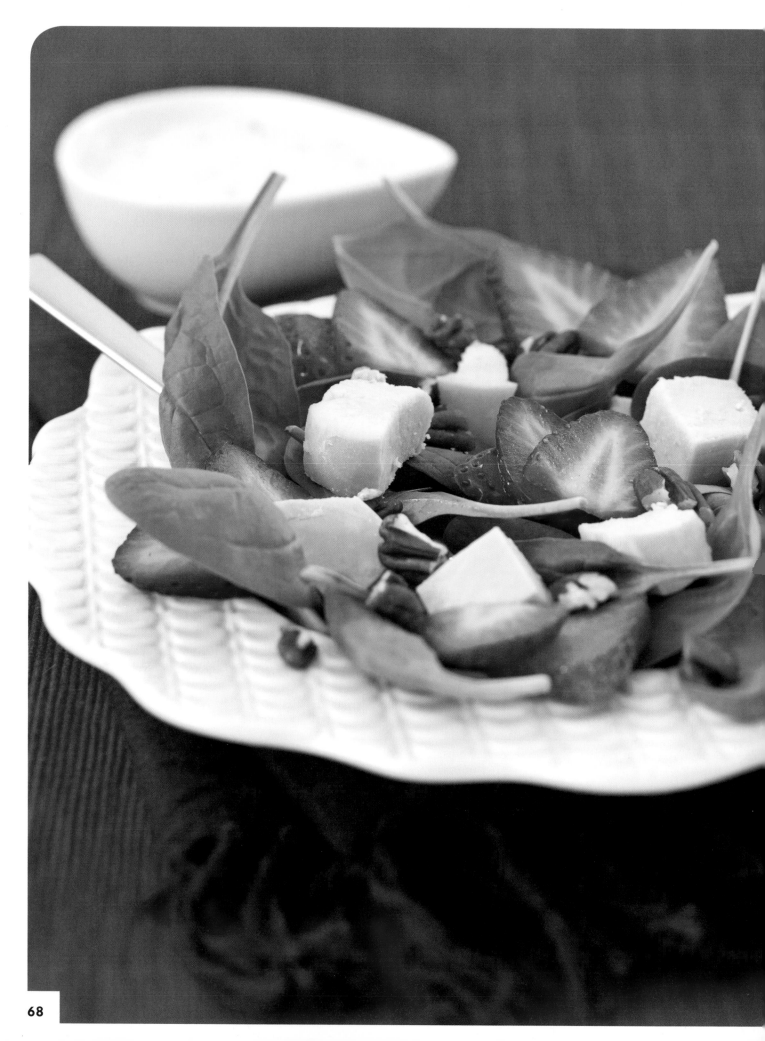

PREP TIME	COOK TIME	SERVES		CALORIES	FAT	PROTEIN	CARBS	FIBER
20 mins	none	4		185	9g	15.5g	13g	3g

STRAWBERRY SPINACH SALAD WITH CHICKEN

"This spinach salad is tossed with fresh strawberries and diced chicken before being topped with chopped pecans and a creamy poppy seed dressing. The dressing has a nice tartness to offset the sweet strawberries."

YOU WILL NEED

1 (9-ounce) package fresh spinach leaves

1 ½ cups strawberries, sliced

1 cup cooked chicken, diced

¼ cup nonfat plain Greek yogurt

1 tablespoon lemon juice

1 tablespoon light agave nectar (may use honey)

1 tablespoon poppy seeds

1 tablespoon canola oil

salt to taste

2 tablespoons chopped pecans

1 Place spinach leaves, strawberries, and diced chicken in a large serving bowl.

2 In a separate bowl, whisk together yogurt, lemon juice, agave nectar, poppy seeds, and canola oil to create the dressing. Season with salt to taste.

3 Drizzle dressing over the salad in the bowl and toss all gently to fully dress. Top with chopped pecans and serve immediately.

CHOOSE THIS!

Strawberries are filled with anthocyanins that not only provide their flush red color but also serve as potent antioxidants that have been shown to help protect the body's cells from free radical damage. This makes these delicious little berries a heart protecting, anti-inflammatory, and possibly even cancer preventing fruit all rolled into one.

LETTUCE EAT SALAD

APPLE CRANBERRY SPINACH SALAD

"This spinach salad with diced apples, cranberries, and chopped walnuts is a quick and unique lunch that is great served alongside a half sandwich or bowl of soup. Or simply top with grilled chicken for a full meal all on its own."

YOU WILL NEED

1 (9-ounce) package baby spinach leaves

1 Granny Smith apple, diced

¼ cup dried cranberries

¼ cup chopped walnuts

¼ cup olive oil

2 tablespoons red wine vinegar

¼ teaspoon salt

⅛ teaspoon pepper

1 Place spinach leaves, diced apple, dried cranberries, and chopped walnuts in a large serving bowl.

2 In a separate bowl, whisk together olive oil, red wine vinegar, salt, and pepper to create a quick vinaigrette.

3 Drizzle dressing over the salad in the bowl and toss all gently to fully dress. Serve immediately.

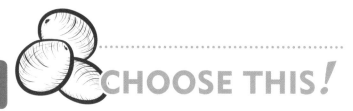

CHOOSE THIS!

Cranberries, including the dried cranberries in this recipe, are very high in antioxidants that can prevent free-radical damage to cells. In addition, they are very well known for their anti-bacterial hippuric acid that can help keep urinary tract infections at bay.

CHICKEN AND AVOCADO SALAD

"Instead of using a prepared dressing that may include less healthy oils, this salad with chicken and avocado is simply dressed in a light drizzle of extra-virgin olive oil and grapefruit juice."

YOU WILL NEED

1 (8-ounce) package chopped romaine lettuce

12 ounces cooked chicken, shredded or sliced

1 pint cherry tomatoes, cut in half

1 avocado, sliced

¼ cup crumbled feta cheese

¼ cup fresh cilantro, chopped

2 tablespoons extra-virgin olive oil

¼ cup grapefruit juice

salt and pepper

1 Divide lettuce equally between 4 large salad bowls.

2 Top each salad with an equal amount of cooked chicken, cherry tomatoes, sliced avocado, feta cheese, and cilantro.

3 Drizzle olive oil and grapefruit juice lightly over each salad. Lightly sprinkle with salt and pepper and serve immediately.

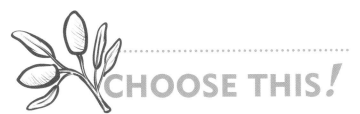

CHOOSE THIS!

Olive Oil is rich in healthy monounsaturated fat (the good fat!) and polyphenols that may have antioxidant qualities. Choose cold-pressed extra virgin olive oil for the oil with the richest flavor and polyphenol content. Also look for dark or paper-covered bottles, as exposure to light can actually affect the oil's flavor and health benefits.

LETTUCE EAT SALAD

GREEK TUNA SALAD

"This tuna salad is mixed with classic Mediterranean ingredients like artichoke hearts, cucumber, tomatoes, and feta cheese for a lunch that is not just high in protein but also entirely unique."

YOU WILL NEED

1 (15.5-ounce) can cannellini beans, drained and rinsed

14 ounces tuna packed in water, drained

½ cup marinated artichoke heart quarters, drained

½ cup diced cucumber

2 Roma tomatoes, diced

1 (10-ounce) package mixed salad greens

3 tablespoons olive oil

salt and pepper

¼ cup crumbled feta cheese

1 In a mixing bowl, gently fold together cannellini beans, tuna, artichoke hearts, cucumber, and tomatoes.

2 Divide mixed salad greens across 4 serving plates.

3 Top salad greens on each plate with a large scoop of the bean and tuna mixture.

4 Drizzle each salad with olive oil and then sprinkle with salt and pepper.

5 Sprinkle each salad with an equal amount of the feta cheese before serving.

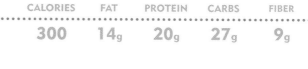

CHOOSE THIS!

Cannellini Beans make this salad distinctively Greek while loading it up with a healthy 9 grams of fiber per serving. This is about ⅓ of your daily recommended amount of fiber, which is a recommendation that far too few people actually meet. These delicious beans also offer a very good amount of calcium, iron, and folate.

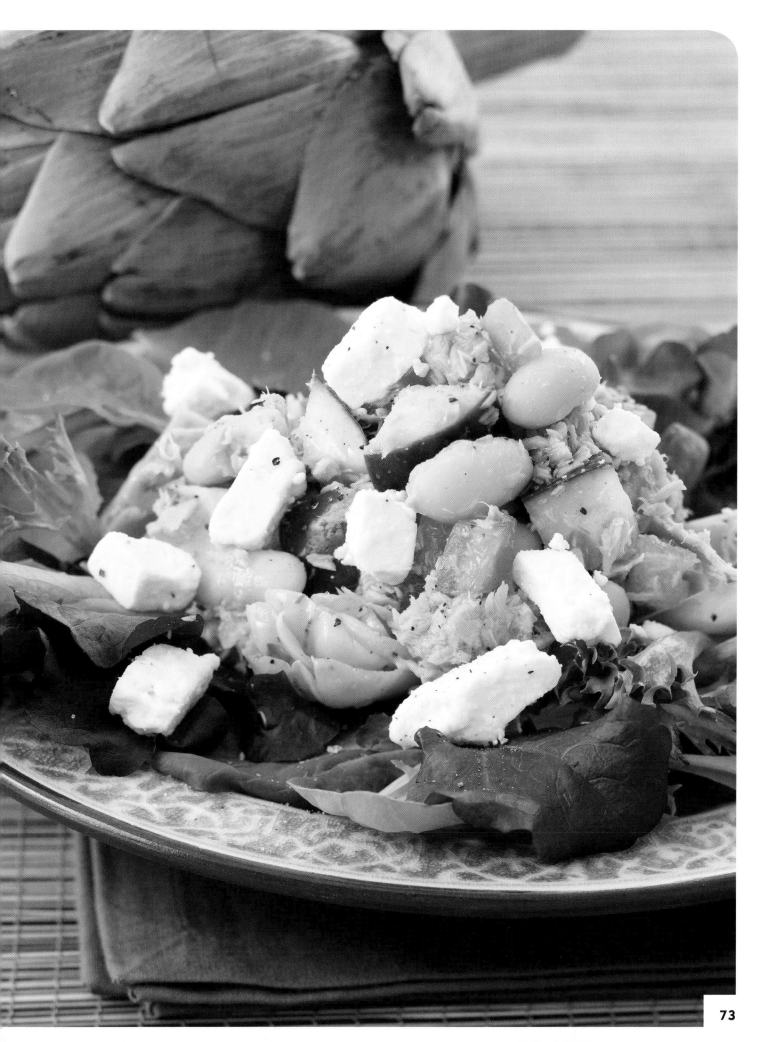

SOUTHWESTERN QUINOA SALAD

"This southwestern salad is made with amazing high-protein quinoa, which is an edible seed that is similar to pearled wheat or tiny grains of rice."

YOU WILL NEED

1 ½ cups water

1 cup dry quinoa

¼ teaspoon salt

1 (15-ounce) can black beans, drained and rinsed

1 cup diced tomatoes

¼ cup diced red onion

½ cup loosely packed fresh cilantro leaves, chopped

juice of 1 lime

3 tablespoons olive oil

salt to taste

1 Place water, quinoa, and salt in a large sauce pan over high heat and bring up to a boil.

2 Cover and let boil 1 minute before reducing heat to low. Let simmer on low 15 minutes.

3 Remove quinoa from heat and let sit 5 minutes.

4 Add all remaining ingredients and stir to combine.

5 Season with salt to taste before serving warm, room temperature, or chilled.

CHOOSE THIS!

Quinoa is a great gluten-free grain-like edible seed usually sold in the pasta aisle in little green boxes. An excellent plant-based source of protein, quinoa actually provides all nine essential amino acids. Look for a box that says that the quinoa is pre-rinsed or simply let regular quinoa soak in water 15 minutes, drain, and rinse before cooking.

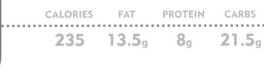

CALORIES	FAT	PROTEIN	CARBS	FIBER
235	13.5g	8g	21.5g	2g

COUSCOUS SALAD

"This Italian-influenced couscous salad includes a colorful mix of red bell pepper, yellow corn, green onions, and spinach. I like to serve this warm, but it is just as good as a chilled picnic salad."

YOU WILL NEED

⅓ cup pine nuts

3 cups cooked couscous (see step 2)

1 tablespoon olive oil

3 green onions, thinly sliced

½ cup diced red bell pepper

1 cup frozen corn kernels

1 cup chopped spinach leaves

1 cup diced fresh mozzarella cheese

⅓ cup prepared pesto sauce

salt and pepper

CHOOSE THIS!

Couscous is made by rolling and shaping moistened semolina wheat and then coating it with finely ground wheat flour. As a result of going through this process, couscous cooks very quickly, making it the perfect thing to prepare in a pinch. Whole wheat couscous is best as it will provide more nutrients and fiber.

1 Preheat oven to 400 degrees F. Place pine nuts on a sheet pan and bake for 5-6 minutes, tossing halfway through. Cook just until the pine nuts are golden brown (toasted) and very fragrant.

2 Prepare couscous according to the package directions. Preparations vary from brand to brand but usually involve a ratio of 2 parts water to 1 part couscous. To prepare 3 cups cooked, start with about 1 ¼ cups of dry.

3 Heat olive oil in a large skillet over medium heat. Add the green onions and diced bell pepper and sauté for 3 minutes.

4 Add the frozen corn to the pan and sauté 1 additional minute before adding the couscous. Stir until the couscous is nice and hot.

5 Add the chopped spinach to the pan, stir to combine, and then remove pan from heat.

6 Stir in toasted pine nuts, mozzarella cheese, and pesto sauce. Add salt and pepper to taste and serve hot or chilled.

LETTUCE EAT SALAD

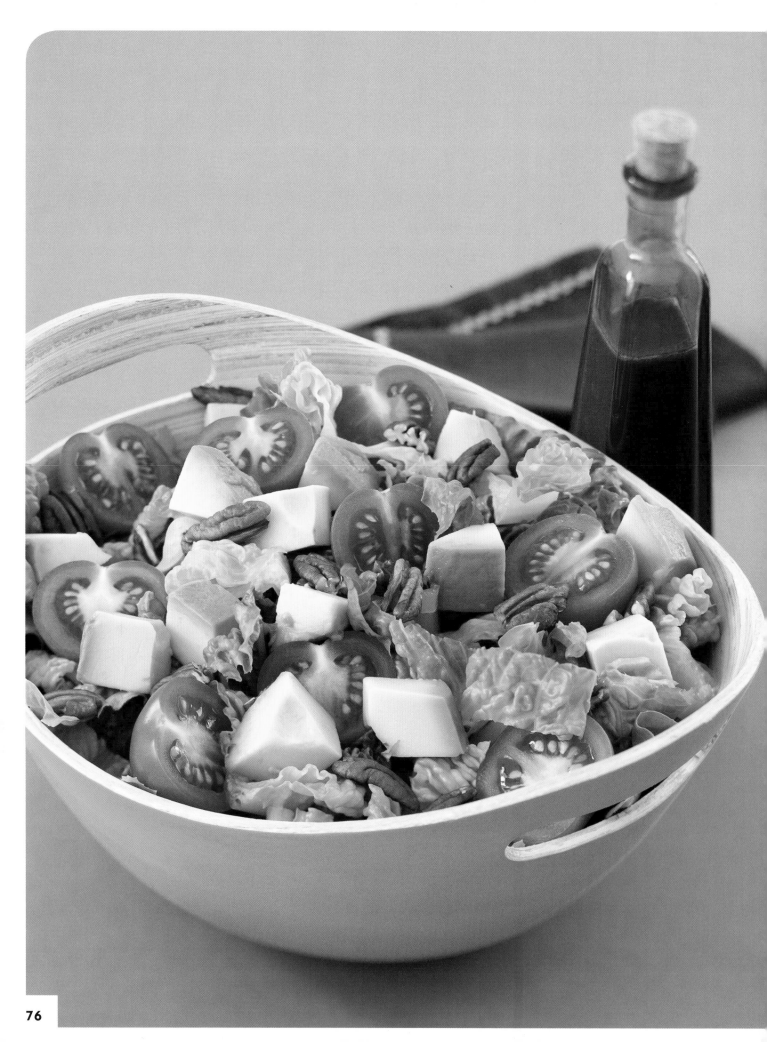

AVOCADO, TOMATO, AND PECAN SALAD

"This family-style salad is the perfect way to start a meal. With the good presence of (monounsaturated) fats found in the avocadoes, olive oil, and pecans, your hunger will be more satisfied and you will be less likely to overeat during the meal to follow."

YOU WILL NEED

⅓ cup olive oil

3 tablespoons balsamic vinegar

1 teaspoon Dijon mustard

½ teaspoon dried dill weed

¼ teaspoon salt

⅛ teaspoon pepper

14 ounces chopped romaine lettuce

1 avocado, peeled and chopped

1 ½ cups cherry tomatoes, halved

¼ cup chopped pecans

1 Whisk together olive oil, balsamic vinegar, Dijon mustard, dill weed, salt, and pepper to create a dressing

2 Add all remaining ingredients to a large serving bowl.

3 Drizzle dressing over the salad in the bowl and toss all gently to fully dress before serving.

CHOOSE THIS!

Avocadoes are an amazingly rich source of healthy monounsaturated fat. They also contain a significant amount of vitamin E and bioactive carotenoids such as lutein and beta-carotene. Carotenoids are fat-soluble, which means that fat must be present to ensure that they are absorbed into the bloodstream—just another reason why the healthy fat in avocadoes is a very good thing!

LETTUCE EAT SALAD

PREP TIME	COOK TIME	SERVES		CALORIES	FAT	PROTEIN	CARBS	FIBER
20 mins	15 mins	6		255	7g	9g	41g	6g

GARDEN FRESH PASTA SALAD

"This pasta salad is not only made with nutritious whole wheat penne pasta, but it's also absolutely brimming with fresh veggies that nourish and detoxify the body."

YOU WILL NEED

8 ounces whole wheat penne pasta

1 cup diced celery

½ cup shredded carrots

1 small cucumber, peeled and diced

1 red bell pepper, diced

6 green onions, thinly sliced

1 cup cherry tomatoes, quartered

¼ cup fresh basil leaves, chopped

2 tablespoons olive oil

2 tablespoons red wine vinegar

¼ teaspoon salt

⅛ teaspoon pepper

¼ cup grated Parmesan cheese

1 Boil pasta according to the package directions, and then drain and rinse under cold water to stop the cooking process.

2 Place cooked pasta in a large serving bowl and top with celery, carrots, cucumber, bell pepper, green onions, cherry tomatoes, and basil.

3 In a separate bowl, whisk together olive oil, red wine vinegar, salt, and pepper to create a quick vinaigrette.

4 Drizzle dressing and Parmesan cheese over the pasta salad in the bowl and toss all gently to fully combine.

5 Chill for at least 30 minutes before serving to let the flavors combine.

CHOOSE THIS!

Basil, especially the fresh basil used in this recipe, is a very good source of vitamin A, which may help prevent free radicals from oxidizing cholesterol in your blood, keeping the cholesterol from building up in your blood vessels.

PREP TIME	COOK TIME	SERVES		CALORIES	FAT	PROTEIN	CARBS	FIBER
20 mins	30 mins	6		295	12g	19g	30g	15.5g

LENTIL SALAD

"Lentils are not just one of the healthiest foods but one of my personal favorites. This salad combines them with tomatoes, walnuts, green onions, and goat cheese for something easy and more than satisfying."

YOU WILL NEED

2 cups water

2 ½ cups chicken broth

1 clove garlic, peeled

1 ½ cups dried lentils

1 tomato, diced

5 green onions, thinly sliced

¼ cup chopped walnuts

¼ cup fresh parsley, chopped

1 clove garlic, minced

2 tablespoons olive oil

3 ounces goat cheese, crumbled

salt and pepper to taste

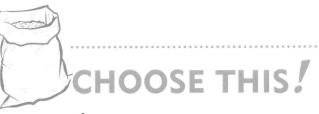

CHOOSE THIS!

Lentils are small, disc-shaped legumes that may seem quite insignificant but are actually one of the most versatile and healthy foods around. They are not only rich in quality protein but also extremely high in dietary fiber as well! Beyond that, they also offer a good amount of potassium and iron.

1 Place water, chicken broth, and the first clove of garlic in a large sauce pan over high heat and bring to a boil.

2 Add lentils to the pot and bring back up to a boil. Cover and reduce heat until just simmering. Cook for 25-30 minutes, until lentils are tender.

3 Remove lentils from heat, drain, and let cool completely before adding to a large serving bowl.

4 Add the tomato, green onions, walnuts, parsley, minced garlic, olive oil, and goat cheese to the lentils in the bowl.

5 Gently toss all to combine. Season with salt and pepper to taste before serving at room temperature or chilled.

ORZO AND TURKEY SALAD WITH CHERRIES

"This chilled salad makes a high-protein and delicious alternative to your typical picnic salads. With turkey, dried cherries, and sage accompanying the orzo pasta, I used to call this my Thanksgiving Leftovers Pasta Salad!"

YOU WILL NEED

8 ounces orzo pasta

½ cup sliced almonds

¾ cup nonfat plain yogurt

2 tablespoons fresh chopped parsley

2 teaspoons fresh chopped sage

¼ teaspoon salt

⅛ teaspoon pepper

1 ½ cups cooked turkey meat, diced (may use chicken)

1 cup diced celery

½ cup dried cherries

½ cup diced red onion

1 Boil orzo according to the package directions. Drain and rinse under cold water.

2 Preheat oven to 350 degrees F. Arrange sliced almonds on a sheet pan and bake 6-8 minutes, just until they smell fragrant. Watch almonds closely, as they burn quickly! Let cool.

3 In a large mixing bowl, combine yogurt, parsley, sage, salt, and pepper.

4 Add the cooked orzo, toasted almonds, and all remaining ingredients to the yogurt mixture and gently fold together until all is combined. Serve chilled.

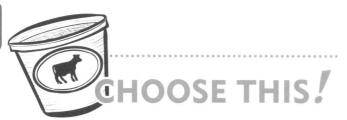

CHOOSE THIS!

Yogurt makes a great low-calorie substitute for mayonnaise in this recipe. High in protein and calcium, yogurt also contains beneficial probiotics that can aid in digestion and inhibit harmful bacteria from growing in your body, boosting immunity.

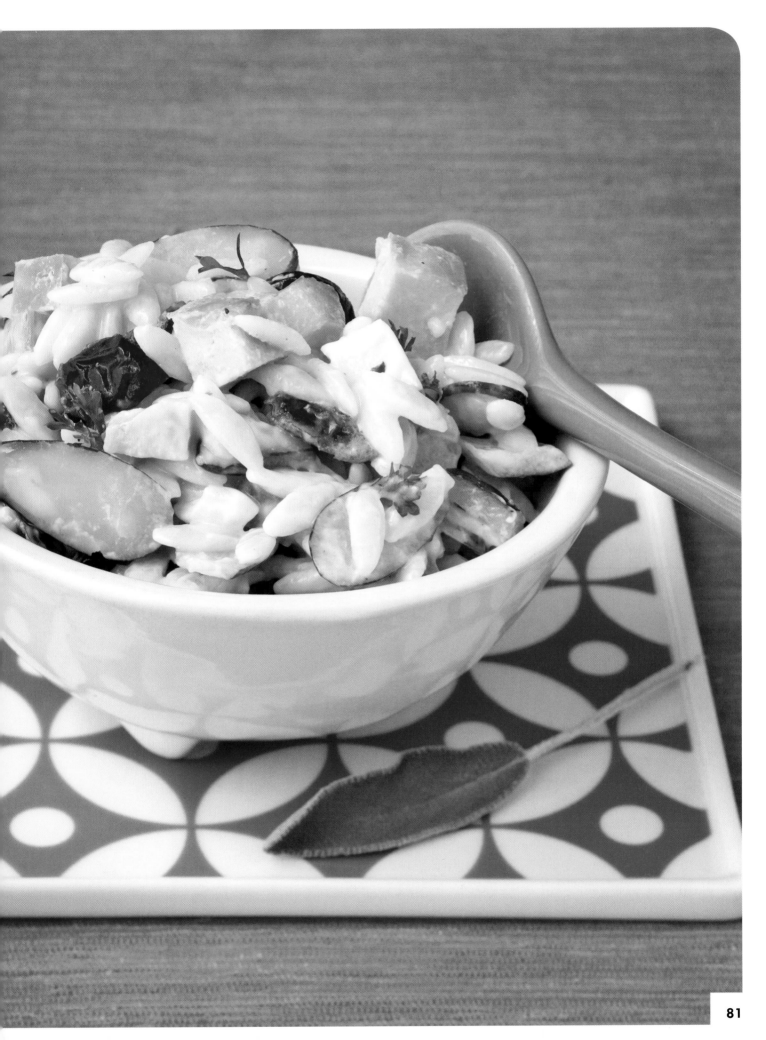

TERIYAKI SALMON SALAD

"Tender salmon fillets make this salad hearty and filling enough to be served as a dinner! The teriyaki dressing lends a great acidity to balance out the fish."

YOU WILL NEED

¼ cup sliced almonds

1 (9-ounce) package chopped lettuce mix

1 cup shredded carrots

3 green onions, thinly sliced

3 tablespoons rice wine vinegar

2 tablespoons reduced-sodium teriyaki sauce

2 teaspoons sesame oil

2 tablespoons light brown sugar

¼ cup olive oil

4 (4-ounce) salmon fillets

salt and pepper

1 Preheat oven to 350 degrees F. Toast sliced almonds by arranging on a sheet pan and baking 6-8 minutes, just until they smell fragrant. Let cool.

2 Divide lettuce, carrots, green onions, and toasted almonds equally between 4 large salad bowls.

3 In a mixing bowl, whisk together rice wine vinegar, teriyaki sauce, sesame oil, brown sugar, and olive oil to create a dressing.

4 Preheat broiler to high. Season salmon with a generous amount of salt and pepper and place on a broiler pan or heavy sheet pan. Place on the second oven rack from the broiler and cook 8-10 minutes, or until flaky.

5 Place 1 cooked salmon fillet atop each salad and serve drizzled with the dressing.

CHOOSE THIS!

Salmon is a great source of essential omega-3 fatty acids, which are anti-inflammatory and play many important roles inside our bodies. These fatty acids are in fact essential, but our bodies do not create them on their own, so they must be present somewhere in our diet.

A PERFECT PEAR SALAD

"Sweet pears and savory bleu cheese make a perfect pair in this spinach salad with a honey balsamic vinaigrette."

YOU WILL NEED

1 (9-ounce) package baby spinach leaves

1 pear, diced

½ cup crumbled low-fat bleu cheese

½ cup sliced celery

1 cup grape tomatoes

¼ cup chopped walnuts

¼ cup olive oil

2 tablespoons balsamic vinegar

2 teaspoons honey

¼ teaspoon minced garlic

⅛ teaspoon salt

⅛ teaspoon pepper

1 Place spinach leaves in a large serving bowl and top with diced pear, crumbled bleu cheese, celery, tomatoes, and walnuts.

2 In a mixing bowl, whisk together olive oil, balsamic vinegar, honey, garlic, salt, and pepper to create a quick vinaigrette.

3 Drizzle dressing over the salad in the bowl just before serving.

CHOOSE THIS!

Pears are a great source of pectin, a fiber that can actually help lower cholesterol levels. This pectin is mainly in the skin of the pear, so be sure to skip the peeler when preparing this salad. Pears are also hypoallergenic, which is why they are a base for many baby foods, as an infant's food allergies may not have beeen discovered.

LETTUCE EAT SALAD

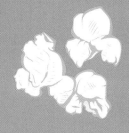

SNACK ATTACK!

• •

"A good, healthy snack can satisfy a late morning or early afternoon hunger attack and keep you from overeating at your next meal."

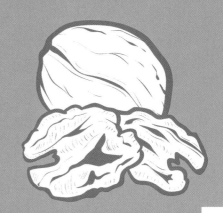

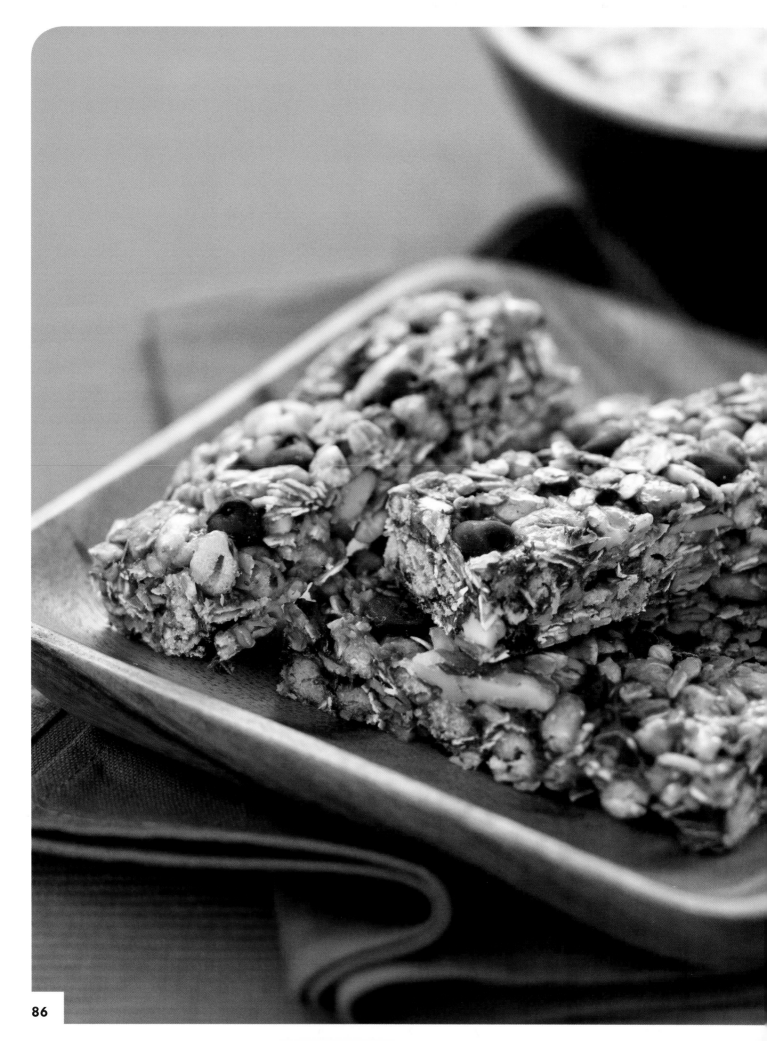

PEANUT BUTTER CUP ENERGY BARS

"We all love the great taste and convenience of energy or granola bars; however, the healthier brands can cost you over $1 a bar. Thankfully, making your own is quite easy and the ingredients purchased can make several large batches of 24 bars each batch."

YOU WILL NEED

1 ½ cups old-fashioned oats
2 ½ cups puffed wheat cereal
½ cup slivered almonds, lightly chopped
¼ cup ground flax seeds
½ cup sunflower seeds
½ cup chopped walnuts
½ cup semisweet chocolate chips
2 tablespoons butter
¾ cup light brown sugar
½ cup natural peanut butter
¾ cup light agave nectar (may use honey)
¼ teaspoon salt
1 teaspoon vanilla extract

CHOOSE THIS!

Agave Nectar is a liquid sweetener extracted from Mexican agave plants. Agave nectar is very low-glycemic, meaning that it will not raise your blood sugar as high as regular sugar and will help keep your metabolism in balance. It is available in the organic or sugar aisle of most grocery stores. Honey can be easily substituted but is much higher on the glycemic index.

1 Line a 13x9 inch pan with wax paper.

2 In a large mixing bowl, combine oats, puffed wheat, almonds, flax seeds, sunflower seeds, walnuts, and chocolate chips.

3 Place butter, brown sugar, peanut butter, agave nectar, and salt in a sauce pan over medium heat and bring to a simmer. Remove from heat and stir in vanilla extract.

4 Pour the hot liquid mixture over the dry ingredients in the mixing bowl and toss all to combine.

5 Spread mixture into the wax paper-lined pan and then cover with another sheet of wax paper. Press the top sheet of wax paper down firmly (as hard as you can!) to fully compress bars and smooth out their tops.

6 Let cool completely, until hardened. To harden faster: place in freezer for 15 minutes. Remove wax paper and cut into 24 bars to enjoy. I store these in the freezer, as they tend to get soft after a night on the counter. If frozen, simply let thaw 15 minutes before eating.

SNACK ATTACK!

PIZZA POPCORN

"This cheesy popcorn is cooked in olive oil and tossed with oregano and garlic for a pizza parlor taste without the chemicals of processed snacks."

YOU WILL NEED

2 tablespoons olive oil

⅔ cup popcorn kernels

3 tablespoons grated Parmesan cheese

¾ teaspoon dry oregano

¼ teaspoon garlic powder

⅛ teaspoon black pepper

sea salt or fine popcorn salt to taste

CHOOSE THIS!

Oregano gives this snack its potent blast of pizza flavor and while the small amount of dry oregano used here may not be enough to make a big nutritional difference, cooking with oregano is always a smart idea! Oregano is actually loaded with antioxidants shown to prevent cell damage in the body. The herb even has antiseptic qualities making it a natural preservative!

1 Place oil in a stirring popcorn maker, old-fashioned cranked popcorn maker, or heavy pot over medium-high heat.

2 Add popcorn kernels and cook until all are popped. If using a stirring popcorn maker: simply cover with bowl and let pop. If using a cranked popcorn maker: crank continuously as the popcorn pops. If using a heavy pot: cover and shake the pot constantly as the popcorn pops.

3 Combine Parmesan cheese, oregano, garlic powder, and black pepper, and then sprinkle over the popcorn immediately after it has finished popping. Toss all to coat.

4 Add salt to taste and serve immediately. Note: You can also make this with an air popper by adding the dry kernels to the popper and simply drizzling 1 tablespoon of olive oil over the popped popcorn before sprinkling with the seasonings. That said, the results will be better with one of the previously mentioned methods.

MIX AND MATCH TRAIL MIX

"I love to bring a bag of trail mix with me to the gym as a great little pick me up, but store-bought mixes are not always the healthiest. Here, I've presented several ingredients that you can mix and match to make your own well-balanced trail mix."

CHOOSE 1 OF EACH

NUTS

1 ¾ cups mixed nuts

2 cups almonds

1 ¼ cups shelled pistachios

SEEDS

½ cup shelled sunflower seeds

¼ cup flax seeds

½ cup shelled pumpkin seeds

FRUITS

⅔ cup dried apples, chopped

½ cup raisins

⅓ cup dried cranberries

SNACKS

⅔ cup Goldfish crackers

½ cup mini pretzels

½ cup Fiber One cereal

SWEETS (optional)

½ cup yogurt-covered raisins

⅓ cup semi-sweet chocolate chips

⅓ cup chopped dark chocolate

Note: Ingredients in **bold** make up my own favorite mix, which is what the nutritional information for this recipe was based on.

1 Choose 1 ingredient from each category and toss together to create your own well balanced trail mix.

2 Store in an airtight container or divide between 12 sealable snack-sized food storage bags for easiest portion-control.

CHOOSE THIS!

Seeds, like those that you can choose from in the seeds category of this recipe, are what really rounds out a healthy trail mix. They are extremely dense with healthy vitamins and minerals, especially when you can find them in their raw form. Sadly, many store bought varieties of trail mix simply don't include seeds at all!

SNACK ATTACK!

POPCORN WITH A KICK

"This, my favorite preparation for popcorn, packs quite a kick. Nobody likes a bland snack and this one is anything but!"

YOU WILL NEED

2 tablespoons canola oil

⅔ cup popcorn kernels

½ teaspoon chili powder

¼ teaspoon ground cumin

½ teaspoon paprika

sea salt or fine popcorn salt to taste

CHOOSE THIS!

Chili Powder is made from chili peppers that contain a substance called **capsaicin**, which not only gives the peppers their characteristic heat, but can also be a potent inhibitor of inflammation in the body. Regularly eating anti-inflammatory foods like chilies and even chili powder can help us defend against chronic diseases linked to inflammation, such as heart disease or type 2 diabetes.

1 Place oil in a stirring popcorn maker, old-fashioned cranked popcorn maker, or heavy pot over medium-high heat.

2 Add popcorn kernels and cook until all are popped. If using a stirring popcorn maker: simply cover with bowl and let pop. If using a cranked popcorn maker: crank continuously as the popcorn pops. If using a heavy pot: cover and shake the pot constantly as the popcorn pops.

3 Combine chili powder, cumin, and paprika, and then sprinkle over the popcorn immediately after it has finished popping. Toss all to coat.

4 Add salt to taste and serve immediately. Note: You can also make this with an air popper by adding the dry kernels to the popper and simply drizzling 1 tablespoon of canola oil over the popped popcorn before sprinkling with the seasonings. That said, the results will be better with one of the previously mentioned methods.

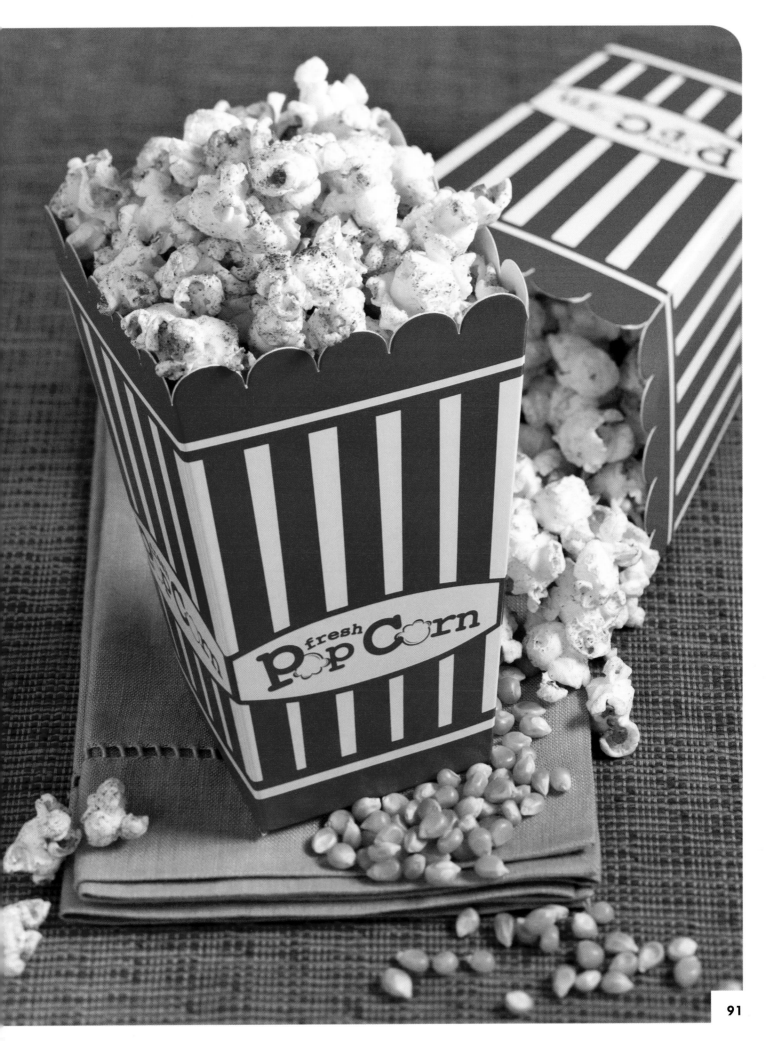

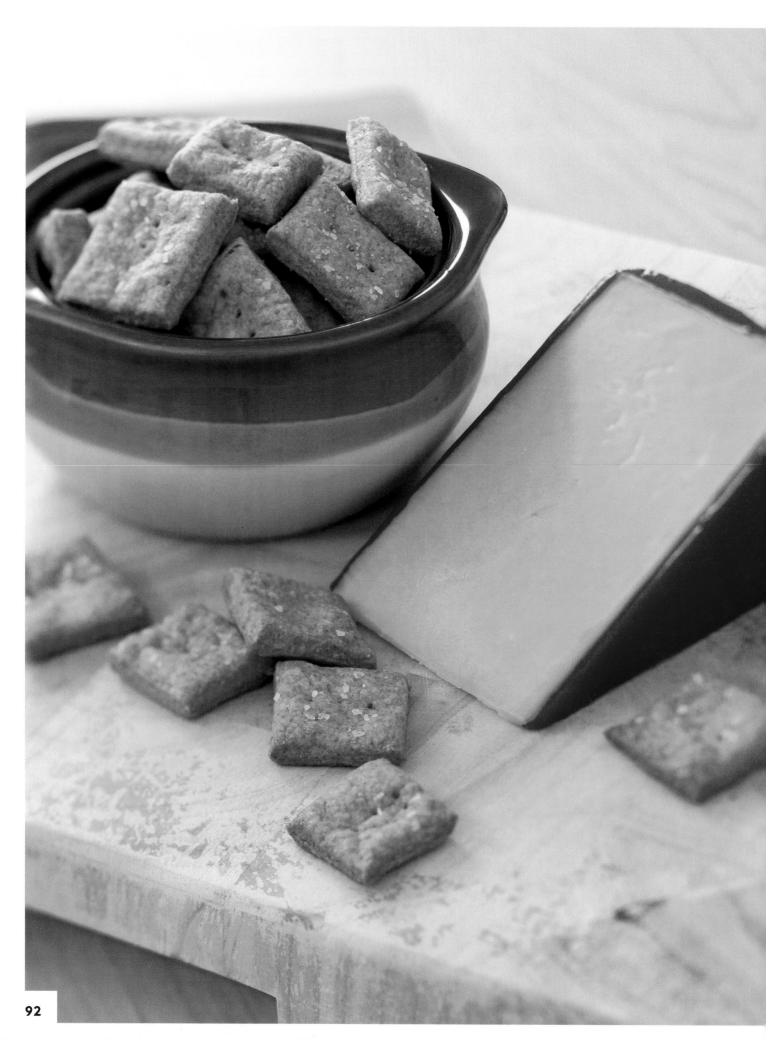

PREP TIME	COOK TIME	SERVES		CALORIES	FAT	PROTEIN	CARBS	FIBER
20 mins	20 mins	8		165	10.5g	5g	12.5g	0.5g

HOMEMADE CHEESE CRACKERS

"Making crackers from scratch is one of those things that makes you feel pretty darn accomplished at the end of the day. Not only are these particular crackers deliciously cheesy, but they also pack in a pretty good amount of whole grains to boot!"

YOU WILL NEED

4 tablespoons butter, softened

1 cup shredded sharp Cheddar cheese

1 cup whole wheat flour

2 tablespoons warm water

¼ teaspoon baking powder

¼ teaspoon onion powder

¼ teaspoon paprika

¼ teaspoon salt

coarse salt, optional

CHOOSE THIS*!*

Whole Grains, like those in the whole wheat flour in this recipe, are much higher in vitamins, minerals, fiber, and antioxidants than refined or "white" grains. Studies have shown that eating more whole grains may help with weight management and reduce the risk of heart disease, cancer, and diabetes.

1 Preheat oven to 350 degrees F.

2 In a large mixing bowl, whisk the softened butter until smooth and then fold in shredded Cheddar cheese.

3 Add all remaining ingredients, except coarse salt, to the bowl and knead until a thick dough is formed.

4 Lay out a long sheet of parchment paper and place dough on top, pressing down to flatten. Cover with an additional sheet of parchment paper. Use a rolling pin over top of the parchment paper to roll the dough out to a thickness of about ⅛ of an inch.

5 Discard top sheet of parchment paper and slice the rolled-out dough into 1-inch squares. Transfer cut squares off of the parchment paper and onto a large sheet pan. Pierce each with a fork and sprinkle with coarse salt, if desired.

6 Bake 15-20 minutes, or until golden brown. Let cool on pan before serving.

SNACK ATTACK!

CALORIES	FAT	PROTEIN	CARBS	FIBER
115	1.5$_g$	8$_g$	18$_g$	9$_g$

BAKED LENTIL SNACKS

"Somewhat spicy and very addictive, these little fiber-packed lentils are baked until all of their moisture cooks out of them, leaving behind a very crunchy snack food that is similar to half-popped popcorn kernels."

YOU WILL NEED

1 ¼ cups lentils

2 teaspoons olive oil

1 teaspoon salt

¼ teaspoon chili powder

¼ teaspoon onion powder

¼ teaspoon garlic powder

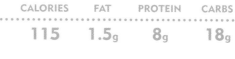

CHOOSE THIS!

Lentils are small disc-shaped legumes that may seem quite insignificant but are actually one of the most versatile and healthy foods around. They are not only rich in quality protein but also extremely high in dietary fiber as well! Beyond that, they also offer a good amount of potassium and iron.

1 Place lentils in a large pot of water over high heat and bring up to a boil. Cover, reduce heat to low, and simmer 12 minutes.

2 Rinse cooked lentils under cold water, drain well, and then pat with paper towels to catch any remaining moisture.

3 Preheat oven to 425 degrees F. In a large mixing bowl, toss lentils in olive oil, salt, chili powder, onion powder, and garlic powder.

4 Spread the coated lentils out in a thin layer on a large sheet pan and bake 30 minutes, shaking the pan halfway through to move them around. Let cool 5 minutes before enjoying.

KETTLE CORN

"This recipe is proof that you don't actually need a giant copper kettle to get all of the salty/sweet flavor of carnival Kettle Corn at home. For the truest recreation of this delicious treat, look for extra-fine salt, which is usually sold in the popcorn section under the name 'popcorn salt.'"

YOU WILL NEED

2 tablespoons canola oil

⅔ cup popcorn kernels

3 tablespoons sugar

sea salt or fine popcorn salt to taste

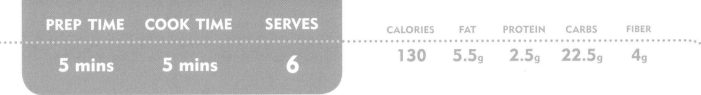

CHOOSE THIS!

Popcorn is actually a whole grain food that (when it isn't smothered in butter) can be a wonderful alternative to high-fat snack foods. Popcorn is very high in heart-healthy fiber that can not only aid in digestion, but also lower cholesterol.

1 Place oil in a stirring popcorn maker, old-fashioned cranked popcorn maker, or heavy pot over medium-high heat.

2 Once oil is hot, add popcorn kernels and sprinkle with sugar.

3 Cook until all kernels are popped. If using a stirring popcorn maker: simply cover with bowl and let pop. If using a cranked popcorn maker: crank continuously as the popcorn pops. If using a heavy pot: cover and shake the pot constantly as the popcorn pops.

4 Add salt to taste and serve immediately.

SNACK ATTACK!

HOMEMADE APPLE CHIPS

"Making your own apple chips at home is actually quite easy, and not only are they far less expensive than the store-bought variety, but they also contain no added oils or fat. Try experimenting with different varieties of apple to find your favorite!"

YOU WILL NEED

2 large apples

2 tablespoons sugar

1 teaspoon ground cinnamon

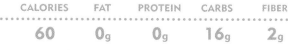

CHOOSE THIS!

Apples are one of the richest sources of fruit pectin, a natural fiber that can help cleanse bad cholesterol from your bloodstream. Many recent studies have also suggested that the rich vitamin and mineral content of apples may provide protection from several major types of cancer.

1 Preheat oven to 215 degrees F. Line 2 large sheet pans with parchment paper.

2 Core apples, if desired. This is not entirely necessary, as the apple will get crisp enough to eat core and all.

3 Use a mandolin or very sharp knife to cut whole apples into ⅛-inch slices. If you chose not to core the apples, shake off any seeds from the slices. Arrange slices in a single layer on the lined sheet pans.

4 Combine sugar and cinnamon, and sprinkle over all sliced apples.

5 Bake 2 hours before turning the oven off, leaving the apples still inside. Let apples sit in the warm oven overnight.

6 Apples should be very crisp. If not, you can turn the oven back up to 200 degrees F. and continue baking until they are. Store in an airtight container.

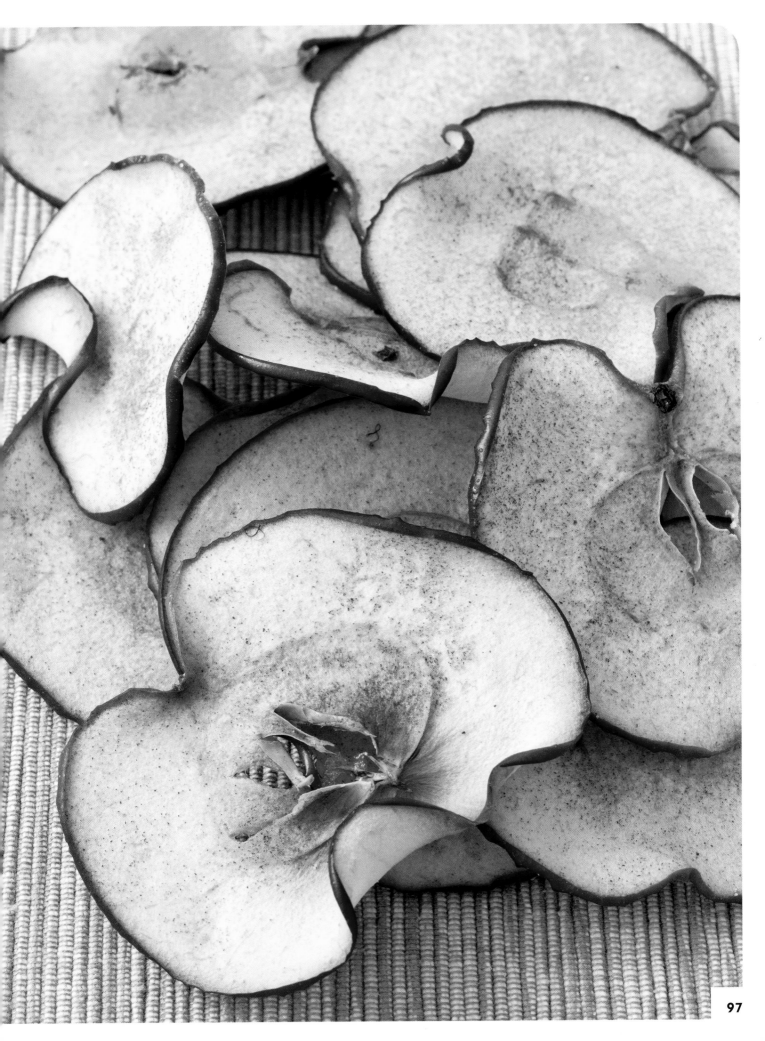

PREP TIME	COOK TIME	SERVES		CALORIES	FAT	PROTEIN	CARBS	FIBER
5 mins	15 mins	12		110	8.5g	3.5g	7g	2g

SWEET AND SALTY ALMONDS

"Much like kettle corn or honey roasted peanuts, these sweet and savory roasted almonds are appropriate as either a snack or a dessert."

YOU WILL NEED

2 cups natural almonds

1 tablespoon light agave nectar (may use honey)

2 teaspoons canola oil

1 tablespoon water

¼ teaspoon ground cinnamon

1 ½ tablespoons sugar

½ teaspoon salt

1 Preheat oven to 325 degrees F. Line a sheet pan with parchment paper.

2 In a mixing bowl, toss together almonds, agave nectar, canola oil, water, and cinnamon until almonds are fully coated.

3 Spread coated almonds in a single layer on the lined sheet pan and bake 15 minutes, stirring halfway through.

4 Remove almonds from oven and toss in sugar and salt before serving. Store in an airtight container.

CHOOSE THIS!

Almonds are regarded as one of the healthiest nuts (though they are technically seeds) with an amazing ability to raise good HDL cholesterol as it lowers bad LDL cholesterol. This "super food" is also high in fiber, magnesium, potassium, and a host of other important vitamins and minerals.

APPLE CINNAMON ENERGY BARS

"I really do enjoy making my own energizing granola bars since it means I'll have a huge batch that I can freeze easily for the perfect workout snack all month long."

YOU WILL NEED

1 ½ cups old-fashioned oats

2 ½ cups puffed wheat cereal

½ cup slivered almonds, lightly chopped

¼ cup ground flax seeds

½ cup sunflower seeds

½ cup chopped walnuts

1 cup dried apples, chopped

2 teaspoons ground cinnamon

2 tablespoons butter

¾ cup light brown sugar

½ cup SoyNut butter

¾ cup light agave nectar (may use honey)

¼ teaspoon salt

½ teaspoon vanilla extract

CHOOSE THIS!

Flax Seeds are typically available in the health food or organic section of major grocery stores (as is the SoyNut butter also featured in this recipe). These mildly nutty seeds are an excellent source of essential omega-3 fatty acids.

1 Line a 13x9 inch pan with wax paper.

2 In a large mixing bowl, combine oats, puffed wheat, almonds, flax seeds, sunflower seeds, walnuts, dried apples, and cinnamon.

3 Place butter, brown sugar, SoyNut butter, agave nectar, and salt in a sauce pan over medium heat and bring to a simmer. Remove from heat and stir in vanilla extract.

4 Pour the hot liquid mixture over the dry ingredients in the mixing bowl and toss all to combine.

5 Spread mixture into the wax paper-lined pan and then cover with another sheet of wax paper. Press the top sheet of wax paper down firmly (as hard as you can!) to fully compress bars and smooth out their top.

6 Let cool completely, until hardened. To harden faster: place in freezer for 15 minutes. Remove wax paper and cut into 24 bars to enjoy. I store these in the freezer, as they tend to get soft after a night on the counter. If frozen, simply let thaw 15 minutes before eating.

SNACK ATTACK!

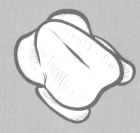

PROTEIN PACKED POULTRY

"Poultry is not only a versatile source of lean protein, but it's also pretty easy on the pocketbook. I like to think that these recipes showcase that versatility in spades."

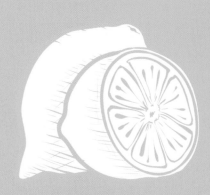

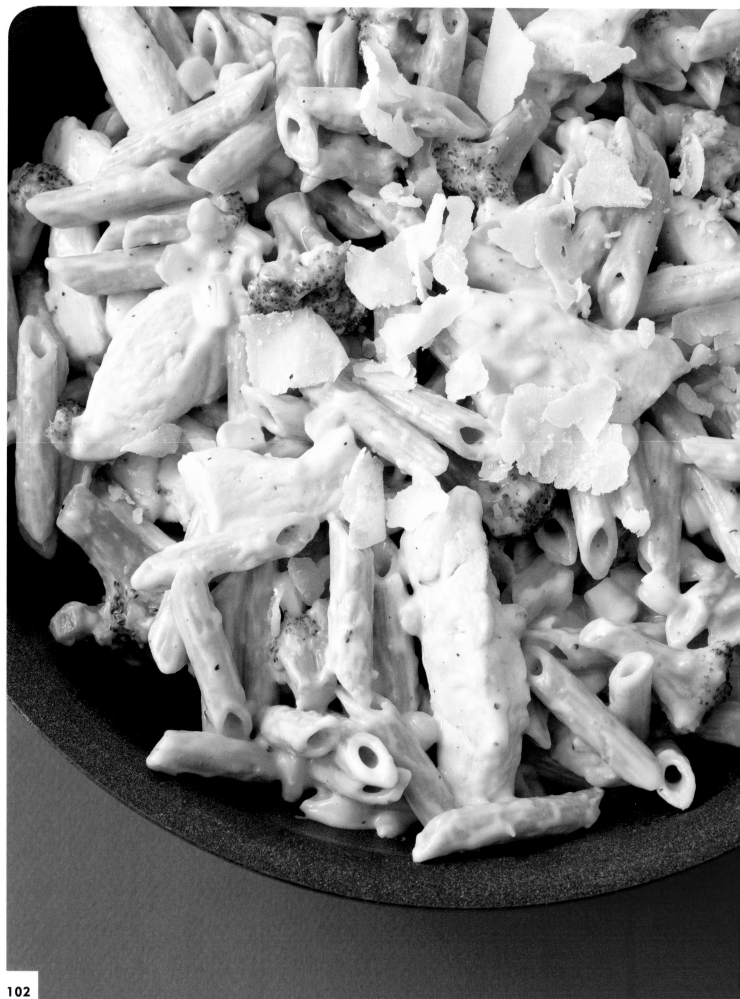

SKILLET CHICKEN ALFREDO

"This hearty, complete skillet meal includes chicken, broccoli, corn, and whole wheat pasta in a creamy Alfredo sauce and still comes in with less than 10 grams of fat!"

YOU WILL NEED

8 ounces whole wheat penne pasta

2 teaspoons olive oil

1 pound boneless, skinless chicken breasts, cut into ¼-inch thick strips

1 tablespoon light butter

2 cups frozen baby broccoli florets

1 cup frozen corn kernels

2 teaspoons minced garlic

1 tablespoon all-purpose flour

1 cup fat-free evaporated milk

2 ounces fat-free cream cheese

⅓ cup grated Parmesan cheese

¼ teaspoon salt

⅛ teaspoon pepper

CHOOSE THIS!

Broccoli is arguably one of the healthiest foods on the planet. Not only does broccoli contain more fiber than whole wheat bread, but it also has more vitamin C than an orange and just as much calcium as a glass of milk!

1 Lightly salt a pot of water and bring up to a boil. Boil whole wheat pasta according to the package directions. Drain well.

2 Meanwhile, as the pasta is cooking, place olive oil in a large skillet over medium-high heat. Add the chicken strips and sauté until browned and cooked throughout, about 5 minutes. Remove from pan and set aside.

3 Add the light butter, frozen broccoli, corn, and garlic to the skillet and sauté 2 minutes.

4 Whisk the flour into the evaporated milk, and add to the skillet along with the cream cheese, Parmesan cheese, salt, and pepper. Stir until the sauce is bubbling and thick.

5 Stir the cooked pasta and chicken into the skillet and sauté an additional 2-3 minutes, just until the broccoli is hot throughout. Serve immediately.

PROTEIN PACKED POULTRY

	PREP TIME	COOK TIME	SERVES		CALORIES	FAT	PROTEIN	CARBS	FIBER
	20 mins	10 mins	4		310	4.5g	35g	33g	8g

CHICKEN WITH BLACK BEAN AND MANGO SALSA

"While this is a very simple preparation of grilled chicken, the savory/ sweet Black Bean and Mango Salsa you serve over the chicken really makes this recipe special."

YOU WILL NEED

1 (15-ounce) can black beans, drained and rinsed

1 mango, peeled and diced

¼ cup finely diced red onion

1 jalapeño, minced

¼ cup fresh cilantro, chopped

1 tablespoon honey

juice of 1 lime

¼ teaspoon salt

4 boneless, skinless chicken breasts

2 teaspoons olive oil

1 teaspoon minced garlic

salt and pepper

1 In a mixing bowl, combine black beans, mango, red onion, jalapeño, cilantro, honey, lime juice, and salt to create the Black Bean and Mango Salsa. Cover and refrigerate until ready to serve.

2 Lightly oil a grill, indoor grill, or grill pan and set to high heat.

3 Toss chicken breasts in olive oil and minced garlic, and then generously season both sides with salt and pepper.

4 Place seasoned chicken breasts onto grill and cook 4-6 minutes on each side, or until slicing into one at its thickest part reveals no pink.

5 Serve grilled chicken topped with the Black Bean and Mango Salsa.

CHOOSE THIS!

Mangos are not only sweet and delicious but are also rich in disease-fighting phytochemicals and vitamins A and C. Look for mangos that feel plump and juicy and not rock hard to ensure proper ripeness.

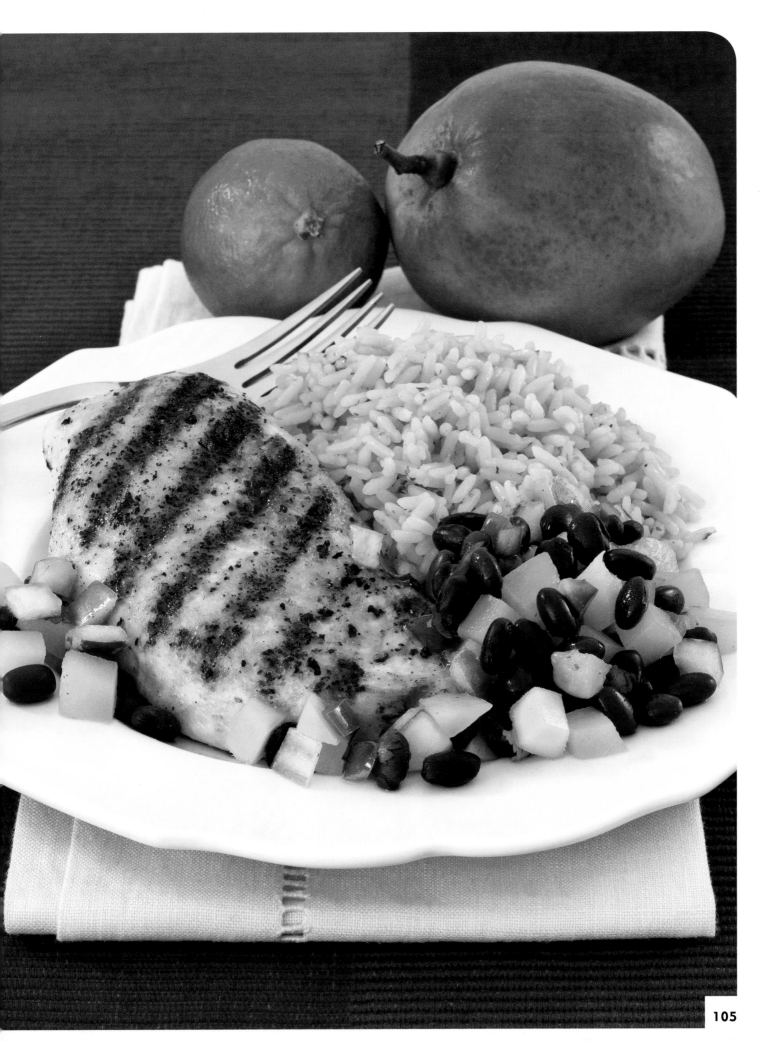

CRISPY BAKED CHICKEN FINGERS

"These baked chicken fingers still retain a hearty crunch thanks to their whole wheat cracker-crumb coating. Serve with your favorite dipping sauces or try them in place of the plain or grilled chicken used in many of the salad recipes in this book."

YOU WILL NEED

nonstick cooking spray

1 cup nonfat plain yogurt

¼ teaspoon salt

⅛ teaspoon pepper

⅛ teaspoon onion powder

1 ½ cups whole wheat Ritz crackers, crushed

1 pound boneless skinless chicken breasts

CHOOSE THIS!

White Meat Chicken helps keep these chicken fingers low in fat and cholesterol. Traditional chicken fingers or nuggets are sometimes made from a combination of white and higher-fat dark meat, not to mention nutritionally empty fillers!

1 Preheat oven to 400 degrees F. Spray a large sheet pan with nonstick cooking spray.

2 In a small bowl, combine yogurt, salt, pepper, and onion powder.

3 Place crushed crackers in a separate bowl.

4 Slice chicken into ½ inch thick strips and then dip into the yogurt mixture.

5 Place each dipped strip of chicken into the cracker crumbs and toss to fully coat. Place the coated strips on the greased baking sheets as you work.

6 Bake 20 minutes, or until cutting into the thickest chicken finger reveals no pink. Serve immediately alongside your favorite dipping sauce.

LEMON AND HERB ROASTED CHICKEN

"This whole roasted chicken is rubbed with dried herbs and fresh lemon juice and stuffed with the actual lemon rinds to guarantee a great flavor throughout every bite."

YOU WILL NEED

1 whole chicken

2 tablespoons olive oil

2 cloves garlic, minced

1 tablespoon dried parsley flakes

1 teaspoon dried rosemary

2 teaspoons dried thyme

¼ teaspoon salt

⅛ teaspoon pepper

1 lemon

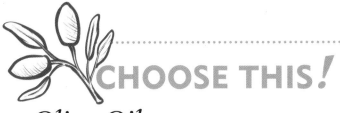

CHOOSE THIS!

Olive Oil is rich in healthy monounsaturated fat (the good fat!) and polyphenols that may have antioxidant qualities. Choose cold-pressed extra virgin olive oil for the oil with the richest flavor and polyphenol content. Also, look for dark or paper-covered bottles, as exposure to light can actually affect the oil's flavor and health benefits.

1 Preheat oven to 400 degrees F.

2 Rinse and pat chicken dry before placing in a shallow roasting pan.

3 In a small bowl, combine olive oil, garlic, parsley, rosemary, thyme, salt, pepper, and the juice of the lemon (reserve the rind) to create an herb rub.

4 Rub the herb rub all over every surface of the chicken and then place breast-side down in the roasting pan. Place lemon rinds into the chicken cavity.

5 Bake 35 minutes before turning the chicken over to breast-side up. Continue baking an additional 30-40 minutes, or until a meat thermometer placed into the center of the thigh registers 180 degrees F.

6 Remove from oven, tent with aluminum foil, and let rest 10 minutes before carving.

PROTEIN PACKED POULTRY

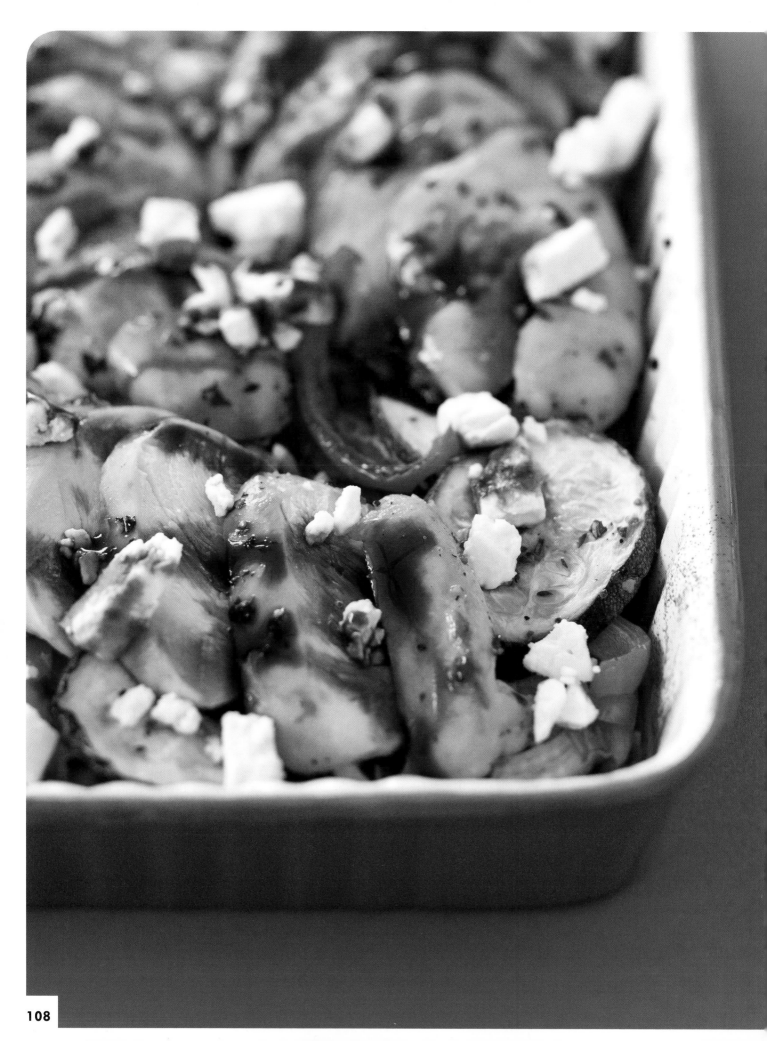

PREP TIME	COOK TIME	SERVES		CALORIES	FAT	PROTEIN	CARBS	FIBER
20 mins	35 mins	4		285	13g	31.5g	11.5g	3g

MEDITERRANEAN CHICKEN AND VEGETABLE BAKE

"These roasted chicken breasts are served over a bed of Mediterranean vegetables and topped with crumbled feta cheese and a drizzle of balsamic vinegar just before serving."

YOU WILL NEED

1 pound boneless, skinless chicken breasts

2 red bell peppers, thinly sliced

2 zucchinis, sliced

1 yellow onion, thinly sliced

2 cloves garlic, minced

2 tablespoons olive oil

1 teaspoon dried oregano

¼ teaspoon salt

⅛ teaspoon pepper

3 ounces crumbled feta cheese

1 tablespoon balsamic vinegar

1 Preheat oven to 375 degrees F.

2 Add all ingredients, except feta cheese and balsamic vinegar, to a large baking dish and toss all to evenly coat with the olive oil, oregano, salt, and pepper.

3 After tossing, arrange chicken breasts atop vegetables in the baking dish and bake 35 minutes, or until cutting into a piece of chicken at its thickest part reveals no pink.

4 Remove from oven, cover with aluminum foil, and let rest for 5 minutes.

5 Remove chicken, slice, and return to the dish. Top with the crumbled feta cheese and drizzle with balsamic vinegar before serving.

CHOOSE THIS!

Zucchini is a great source of folate, potassium, and vitamin A. At only about 25 calories each and with the ability to quickly absorb flavors, zucchini make wonderful "fillers" to help you bulk up any dish with very little caloric or flavor impact.

TURKEY SAUSAGE LASAGNA

"This giant lasagna with fresh spinach and a turkey sausage meat sauce is sure to feed as many people as you can fit around the table!"

YOU WILL NEED

nonstick cooking spray

1 tablespoon olive oil

2 cloves garlic, minced

1 pound ground turkey sausage

2 jars prepared spaghetti sauce

1 (15-ounce) tub low-fat ricotta cheese

4 cups part-skim mozzarella cheese

1 ¾ cups grated Parmesan cheese

1 large egg, beaten

6 basil leaves, chopped

¼ teaspoon salt

⅛ teaspoon pepper

8 ounces dry lasagna noodles

6 ounces fresh spinach leaves

CHOOSE THIS!

Ground Turkey Sausage
is used in this recipe in place of pork sausage or ground beef as it has about ½ of the calories and far lower amounts of saturated fat and cholesterol. "Italian seasoned" ground turkey (sold by Jenny-O) can also be used in this recipe.

1 Preheat oven to 375 degrees F. Spray a 13x9 inch baking dish with nonstick cooking spray.

2 Heat olive oil in a large skillet over medium-high heat. Add the garlic and sauté for 1 minute before adding ground turkey sausage. Cook until sausage is thoroughly browned, breaking it up as it cooks.

3 Cover browned meat with the spaghetti sauce, reduce heat to low, and let simmer 5 minutes.

4 In a mixing bowl, combine ricotta cheese, 1 cup of the mozzarella cheese, ¾ cup of the Parmesan cheese, egg, basil, salt, and pepper.

5 Spread 1 ½ cups of the meat sauce over the bottom of the baking dish.

6 Layer 3 dry noodles over the sauce and top with layers of ⅓ of each of the ricotta cheese mixture, spinach leaves, remaining meat sauce, remaining mozzarella cheese, and remaining Parmesan cheese.

7 Repeat the last step 2 more times to create 2 additional layers. Cover with aluminum foil and bake 60 minutes, uncovering for the last 20. Let sit 15 minutes before slicing.

GREEK CHICKEN PACKETS

"In this recipe, chicken breasts are combined with kalamata olives, Roma tomatoes, feta cheese, olive oil, and herbs for a complete Mediterranean experience in a nice and tidy packet."

YOU WILL NEED

4 boneless, skinless chicken breasts

1 tablespoon olive oil

2 teaspoons Italian seasoning

⅛ teaspoon salt

⅛ teaspoon pepper

5 ounces fresh spinach leaves

2 Roma tomatoes, sliced

1 small red onion, thinly sliced

¼ cup sliced kalamata olives (may use black olives)

½ cup herbed and crumbled feta cheese (may use regular feta)

1 Preheat oven to 375 degrees F. Unroll aluminum foil until the length is roughly equal to the width. Tear out 4 of these large squares and arrange on your counter space.

2 Toss chicken breasts in olive oil, Italian seasoning, salt, and pepper and then place 1 breast in the center of each piece of foil.

3 Arrange an equal amount of the spinach, tomatoes, red onion, olives, and feta cheese over top of each chicken breast.

4 Fold the sides of the aluminum foil in to seal the chicken and toppings into a "packet".

5 Bake packets directly on rack for 25-30 minutes (25 for small chicken breasts).

6 Check for doneness and transfer the contents of each packet to plates before serving. Be careful of hot steam as you open the packets!

CHOOSE THIS!

Kalamata Olives are celebrated for their slightly sweet and entirely rich flavor. If you are watching your sodium, you can look for olives that are packed in vinegar or oil rather than the more traditional (and salty) brine.

PROTEIN PACKED POULTRY

PREP TIME	COOK TIME	SERVES		CALORIES	FAT	PROTEIN	CARBS	FIBER
15 mins	25 mins	8		430	15.5g	20g	53g	7g

PASTA RUSTICO WITH TURKEY SAUSAGE

"This simple and fresh Italian sausage sauté served over whole wheat penne pasta makes a rustic and delicious alternative to heavy, red meat based sauces."

YOU WILL NEED

1 pound whole wheat penne pasta

1 tablespoon olive oil

1 pound Italian turkey sausage links, sliced

1 red onion, thinly sliced

2 red bell peppers, thinly sliced

2 cloves garlic, minced

¾ teaspoon Italian seasoning

3 ounces fresh spinach leaves

¼ teaspoon salt

⅛ teaspoon pepper

¼ cup grated Parmesan cheese

CHOOSE THIS!

Bell Peppers of all colors, but especially the red variety, are loaded with vitamins A and C and several phytochemicals that can help protect cells from damage. Though red bell peppers are nothing more than mature green bell peppers, they are much sweeter and contain as much as 3 times the vitamin C.

1 Bring a large pot of lightly-salted water to a boil. Add pasta and cook 8-10 minutes, just until al-dente. Save ¾ cup of the pasta cooking water before draining!

2 Meanwhile, heat olive oil in a large skillet over medium-high heat. Add sausage and cook until evenly browned and cooked throughout. Remove from pan and set aside.

3 Add onion, peppers, garlic, and Italian seasoning to the empty pan and cook until onions are translucent, about 3-4 minutes.

4 Return sausage to the pan and cook for 2-3 minutes, just until fully reheated throughout. Add spinach, salt, pepper, and reserved pasta water to the pan and immediately remove from heat. Stir until all is combined.

5 Serve the sausage mixture smothered over pasta and topped with the grated Parmesan cheese.

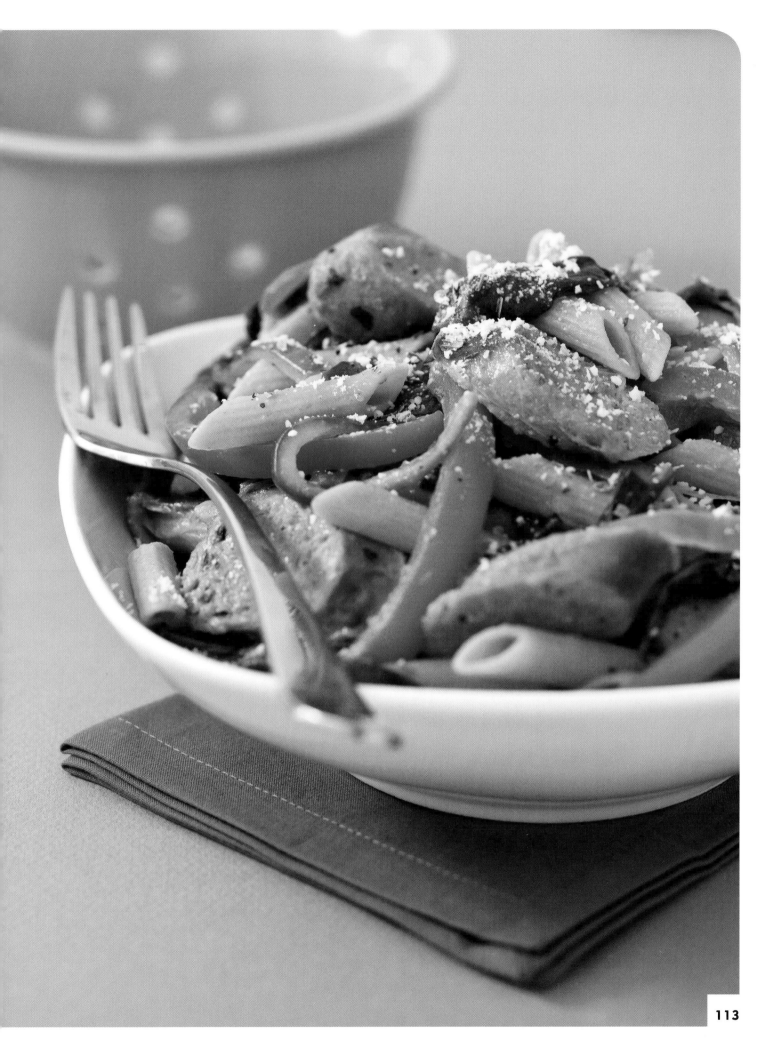

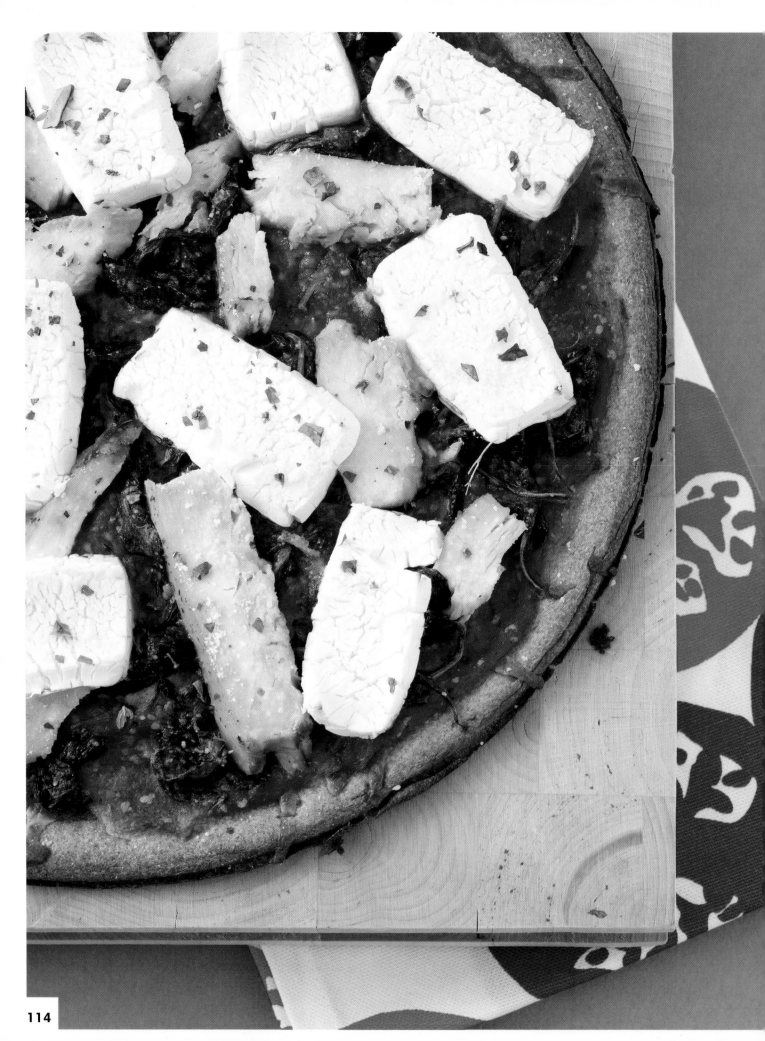

PREP TIME	COOK TIME	SERVES		CALORIES	FAT	PROTEIN	CARBS	FIBER
25 mins	20 mins	4		375	8.5g	28.5g	48g	8g

CHICKEN, SPINACH, AND CREAM CHEESE PIZZA

"This simple pizza topped with chicken, fresh spinach, and cream cheese bakes into a creamy and delicious alternative to traditional mozzarella covered pies."

YOU WILL NEED

1 prepared whole wheat thin pizza crust (such as Boboli brand)

1 cup prepared pizza sauce

1 teaspoon olive oil

2 packed cups fresh spinach leaves

1 (8 or 10-ounce) package cooked Italian chicken strips

1 (8-ounce) package fat-free cream cheese

2 tablespoons grated Parmesan cheese

¼ teaspoon Italian seasoning

CHOOSE THIS!

Spinach is rich in vitamins, minerals, and antioxidants. It also contains choline and inositol, which can prevent hardening of the arteries. When it comes to fresh spinach leaves, baby spinach is softer and best suited for salads due to its higher water content. Regular spinach will release the least water when cooking.

1 Preheat oven to 450 degrees F. Place pizza crust on a large sheet pan and spread pizza sauce over the entire surface.

2 Place olive oil and spinach in a sauté pan over medium heat and sauté just until spinach cooks down. Drain extremely well of excess liquid, being sure to press spinach with a heavy spoon to release additional moisture.

3 Spread cooked and drained spinach and chicken evenly over the surface of the pizza.

4 Slice cream cheese into thin slices and arrange over the other ingredients on the pizza. Sprinkle all with Parmesan cheese and Italian seasoning.

5 Bake 12-14 minutes, just until crust is crispy and cream cheese is hot. Let cool 5 minutes before slicing into 8 slices and serving 2 per portion.

TURKEY PICCATA

"I am always looking for ways to prepare turkey beyond the traditional roasted bird. This recipe for crispy, breaded turkey cutlets in a lemon and caper sauce is traditionally made with chicken (you may substitute chicken if turkey cutlets are unavailable), but I find moist and tender turkey a nice change of pace."

YOU WILL NEED

3 large egg whites, beaten

1 ½ cups whole grain breadcrumbs

salt and pepper

2 pounds turkey cutlets, about ¼ inch thick

¼ cup olive oil

¼ cup lemon juice

1 ½ cups chicken broth

1 tablespoon capers

2 tablespoons fresh chopped parsley

CHOOSE THIS!

Lemons, like most citrus fruits, are abundant with vitamin C. Also, it is commonly used in household cleaning products as its citric acid is a potent disinfectant. These same disinfectant qualities can actually cleanse your stomach and boost your immunity.

1 Preheat oven to 200 degrees F. or use your oven's "warm" setting. Place egg whites and breadcrumbs in 2 separate bowls. Season each with a pinch of salt and pepper.

2 Dip turkey cutlets into egg whites and then into breadcrumbs, fully coating on both sides.

3 Add ½ of the olive oil to a large skillet over medium-high heat. Once hot, add ½ of the breaded turkey cutlets and cook until browned on both sides. Transfer to an oven-safe dish and cover with aluminum foil.

4 Repeat step 3, finishing a second batch with the remaining olive oil and breaded turkey cutlets. Add this batch to the baking dish and re-cover with foil. Place in the warm oven.

5 Create the sauce by adding lemon juice and chicken broth to the skillet you cooked the turkey in, scraping any browned turkey juices into the broth with a spatula. Reduce heat to low and let simmer for 10 minutes, or until the liquid has reduced by about ⅓.

6 Remove sauce from heat and stir in capers.

7 Remove turkey cutlets from oven and serve smothered in the sauce and sprinkled with fresh parsley.

TUSCAN TURKEY SAUSAGE STEW

"This fresh and vibrant stew with a chicken and tomato broth is packed with the protein of turkey sausage and Italian cannellini beans."

YOU WILL NEED

2 tablespoons olive oil

12 ounces Italian turkey sausage links, sliced

1 yellow onion, diced

1 zucchini, diced

2 cloves garlic, minced

½ teaspoon dried oregano

1 (14.5-ounce) can diced tomatoes

1 cup canned cannellini beans, drained and rinsed

6 cups chicken broth

2 cups fresh spinach, chopped

½ cup grated Parmesan cheese

salt and pepper

1 Heat olive oil in a large pot over medium-high heat. Add sliced sausage and sauté until browned on both sides.

2 Add the onion, zucchini, garlic, and oregano to the pot and cook until onions are translucent.

3 Cover with the diced tomatoes, cannellini beans, and chicken broth and bring soup up to a boil. Boil 2 minutes.

4 Reduce heat to low and stir in spinach and Parmesan cheese. Cook 5 additional minutes before seasoning with salt and pepper to taste. Serve hot.

PROTEIN PACKED POULTRY

CHOOSE THIS!

Cannellini Beans are a wonderfully mild white bean that, like most beans and legumes, are a great source of fiber and protein. These Mediterranean beans also offer a very good amount of calcium, iron, and folate.

GRILLED CHICKEN PARMESAN

"I find that, thanks to the grill, this version of Chicken Parmesan made with grilled chicken is actually more flavorful than breaded and deep-fried versions. Serve over whole wheat pasta and alongside a salad for a complete meal."

YOU WILL NEED

4 (6-ounce) boneless, skinless chicken breasts

2 teaspoons olive oil

1 teaspoon minced garlic

¼ teaspoon Italian seasoning

¼ teaspoon salt

⅛ teaspoon pepper

½ cup spaghetti sauce

4 slices provolone cheese

4 large basil leaves

2 tablespoons grated Parmesan cheese

CHOOSE THIS!

Basil, especially the fresh basil used in this recipe, is a very good source of vitamin A, which may help prevent free radicals from oxidizing cholesterol in your blood, keeping the cholesterol from building up in your blood vessels.

1 Lightly oil a grill, indoor grill, or grill pan and set to high heat.

2 Toss chicken breasts in olive oil, minced garlic, Italian seasoning, salt, and pepper.

3 Place seasoned chicken breasts onto grill and cook 4-6 minutes on each side, or until slicing into one at its thickest part reveals no pink.

4 Preheat broiler to high. Transfer grilled chicken breasts to a sheet pan and top each with a large spoonful of spaghetti sauce.

5 Cut each slice of provolone cheese in half and sandwich a basil leaf in between the two halves. Place atop each of the sauced chicken breasts. Sprinkle Parmesan cheese over top all.

6 Broil 3-4 minutes, just until cheese is bubbly and beginning to brown. Serve immediately.

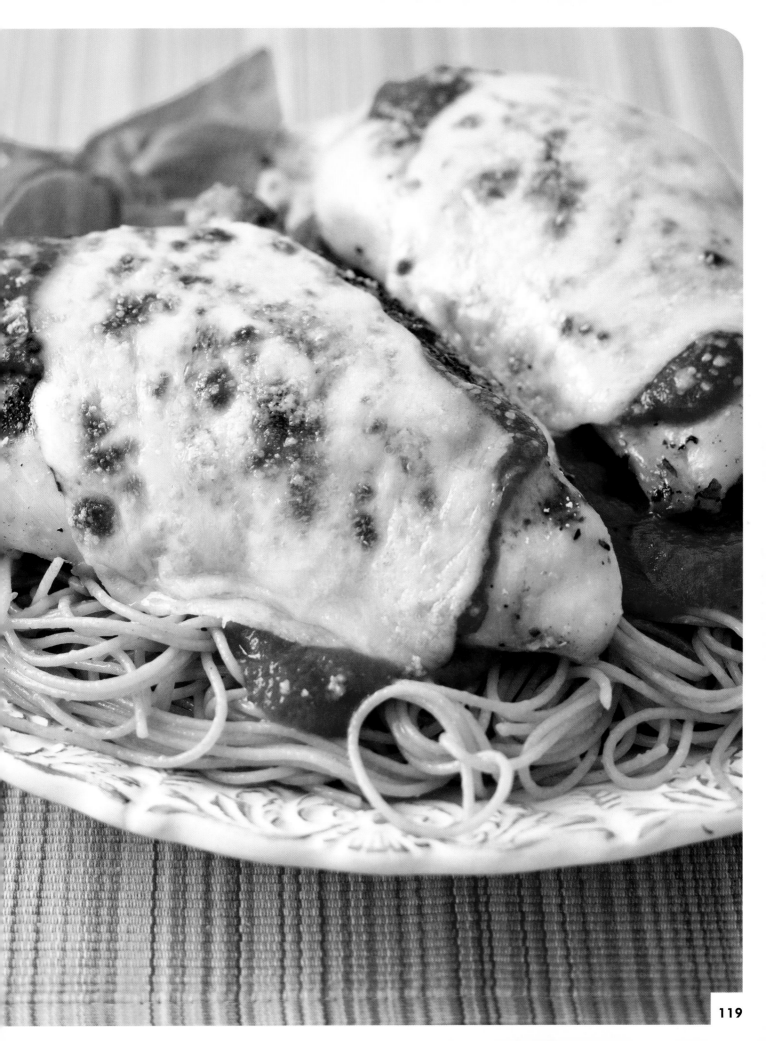

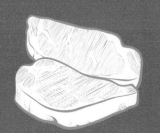

LEAN MEATS

···

"Beef and pork can absolutely have their place in a healthy and active lifestyle; you just have to know the leanest cuts to choose."

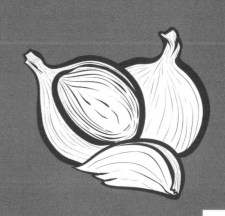

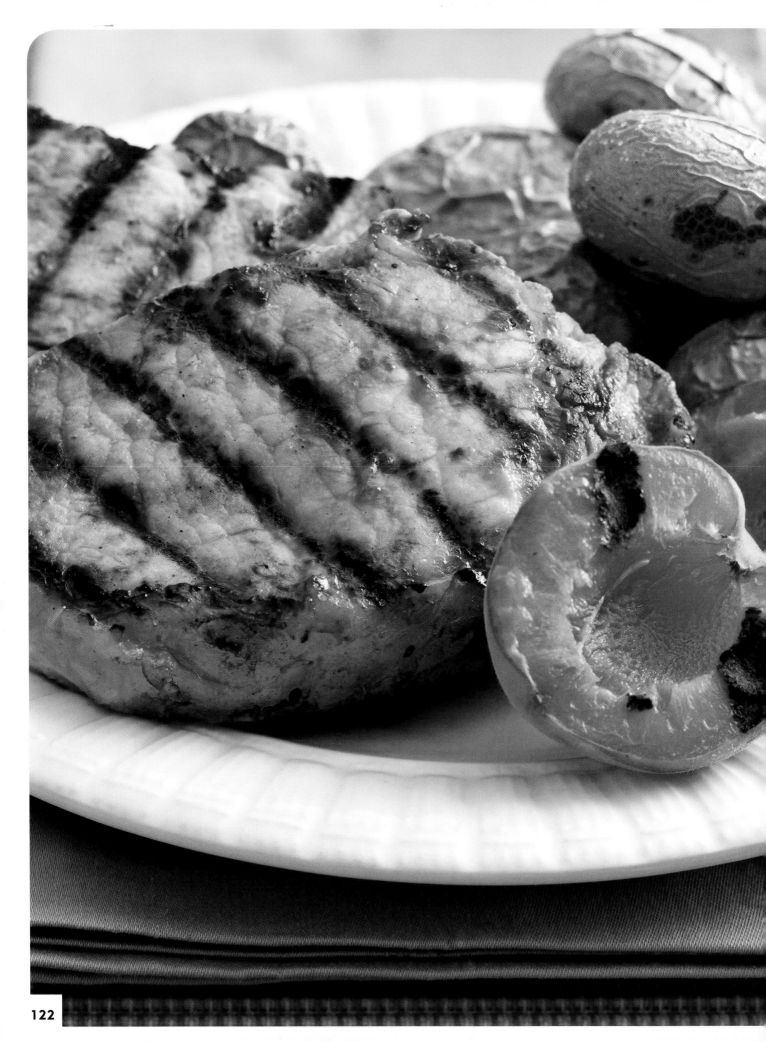

	PREP TIME	COOK TIME	SERVES		CALORIES	FAT	PROTEIN	CARBS	FIBER
	15 mins	20 mins	4		360	10g	45.5g	21.5g	1g

GRILLED APRICOT PORK CHOPS

"Grilled apricot halves make the perfect garnish for these low-fat pork loin chops marinated in a quick marinade of Dijon mustard and jarred apricot preserves."

YOU WILL NEED

½ cup apricot preserves

1 tablespoon Dijon mustard

1 teaspoon minced garlic

¼ teaspoon salt

4 (6-ounce) boneless pork loin chops, about ¾-inch thick

1 tablespoon canola oil

4 apricots, halved and pitted

nonstick cooking spray

1 In a mixing bowl, whisk together apricot preserves, Dijon mustard, minced garlic, and salt to create a marinade.

2 Place pork chops in marinade and toss to coat. Cover and refrigerate for at least 30 minutes to marinate.

3 Lightly oil a grill, indoor grill, or grill pan and set to high heat.

4 Spray the cut side of the apricot halves with nonstick cooking spray.

5 Remove pork chops from marinade and grill 7-8 minutes on each side, or until slicing into one at the thickest point reveals no pink.

6 Place apricots on the grill, cut-side down, and grill 1-2 minutes, just until well-marked. Serve 2 halves alongside each grilled pork chop.

LEAN MEATS

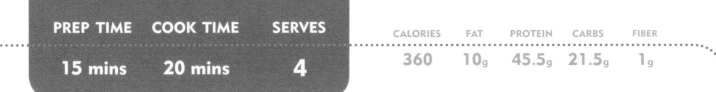

CHOOSE THIS!

Lean Pork is not only tender and delicious but also a very healthy source of high-quality protein. Pork loin and the pork loin chops in this recipe are some of the leanest cuts of pork you can get. Also featured in this book is pork tenderloin, which is actually leaner than chicken breast!

ROSEMARY AND CITRUS PORK TENDERLOIN

"Rosemary and citrus are a perfect combination, especially when used as a marinade for lean pork tenderloin as they are in this recipe. Serve alongside brown rice and my Snappy Peas, recipe page: 156 for a perfectly balanced meal."

YOU WILL NEED

1 pork tenderloin, about 1 ¼ pounds

1 tablespoon olive oil

½ cup orange juice

2 teaspoons fresh chopped rosemary

1 teaspoon lemon juice

2 cloves garlic minced

2 teaspoons light brown sugar

½ teaspoon orange zest

¼ teaspoon crushed red pepper flakes

¼ teaspoon salt

⅛ teaspoon pepper

CHOOSE THIS!

Oranges, as everyone knows, are a wonderful source of vitamin C. Lesser known, however, is their high content of calcium for strong bones, folic acid for a sharp mind, and the same beta-carotene that you find in carrots for healthy eyes.

1 Place pork tenderloin in a food storage container with olive oil, orange juice, rosemary, lemon juice, garlic, brown sugar, orange zest, red pepper flakes, salt, and pepper, tossing all to coat. Cover and refrigerate for 1 hour to marinate.

2 Preheat oven to 450 degrees F. Line a sheet pan with aluminum foil.

3 Remove tenderloin from marinade and place on the lined sheet pan. Use a slotted spoon to capture zest, garlic, and rosemary floating in the marinade and spread over top of the tenderloin.

4 Bake 15-20 minutes, or until a meat thermometer inserted into the thickest part registers 160 degrees F. Let rest under aluminum foil for 10 minutes before slicing to serve.

SPAGHETTI SQUASH WITH MEAT SAUCE

"Spaghetti squash is a (much) more nutritious substitute for high-carbohydrate pasta in this simple dish topped with a homemade meat ragu."

YOU WILL NEED

2 spaghetti squash

2 tablespoons olive oil

1 yellow onion, diced

2 cloves garlic, minced

1 pound extra-lean ground beef

2 (15-ounce) cans tomato sauce

1 bay leaf

2 teaspoons Italian seasoning

1 ½ teaspoons sugar

¼ cup grated Parmesan cheese

salt and pepper

CHOOSE THIS!

Spaghetti Squash is a relatively large squash with stringy pulp that makes a surprisingly great low-calorie and low-carbohydrate substitution for spaghetti and other types of pasta. It has a very mild nuttiness but can easily take on the flavors of anything you top it with.

1 Preheat oven to 400 degrees F. Prick the rind of both spaghetti squash with a fork in several places before placing on a large sheet pan. Bake 1 hour.

2 Meanwhile, heat olive oil in a large skillet over medium-high heat. Add the onion and sauté until translucent.

3 Add the garlic and ground beef to the skillet and thoroughly brown meat, breaking it up as it cooks.

4 Cover browned meat with the tomato sauce, bay leaf, Italian seasoning, and sugar, and then bring up to a boil. Reduce heat to low and simmer 45 minutes.

5 Once squash is baked, remove from oven and let cool enough to handle. Cut both squash in half, discard seeds, and use a fork to scrape the spaghetti strands of the pulp into a large bowl. Toss strands with Parmesan cheese and a pinch of salt and pepper.

6 Season cooked meat sauce with salt and pepper to taste before serving over the seasoned spaghetti squash.

LEAN MEATS

PREP TIME	COOK TIME	SERVES		CALORIES	FAT	PROTEIN	CARBS	FIBER
25 mins	12 mins	6		190	11g	19.5g	2g	1g

STUFFED FLANK STEAK

"This spinach and Parmesan cheese stuffed flank steak is rolled up and sliced into pinwheels for an awe-inspiring presentation."

YOU WILL NEED

1 teaspoon olive oil

1 (9-ounce) bag fresh spinach leaves

¼ cup finely diced red bell pepper

2 cloves garlic, minced

⅛ teaspoon salt

⅛ teaspoon pepper

½ cup grated or shredded Parmesan cheese

1 pound flank steak

baking twine, soaked in water

3 teaspoons olive oil

CHOOSE THIS!

Spinach is rich in vitamins, minerals, and antioxidants. It also contains choline and inositol, which can help prevent hardening of the arteries. When it comes to fresh spinach leaves, baby spinach is softer and best suited for salads due to its higher water content. Regular spinach will release the least water when cooking.

1 Place the 1 teaspoon olive oil, spinach, red bell pepper, garlic, salt, and pepper in a sauté pan over medium heat and sauté just until spinach cooks down. Drain extremely well of excess liquid. Stir in Parmesan cheese.

2 Set oven rack in its highest position and preheat broiler to high. Line a heavy sheet pan with aluminum foil.

3 Lay flank steak on a cutting board with the grain of the steak running horizontally. Carefully "butterfly" steak by slicing from left to right, stopping about 1 inch from the steak's edge. You should now be able to unfold the steak into 1 large piece.

4 Lay out 4 lengths of baking twine on the cutting board and then place the butterflied steak over top of them. Spread the spinach mixture over top the entire surface of the steak.

5 Roll steak into a long, tight pinwheel and tie baking twine to hold that shape. Rub the outside with olive oil and season generously with salt and pepper.

6 Place on lined sheet pan and broil 10–15 minutes, flipping halfway through, until a thermometer registers 145 degrees F for medium-rare (160 for medium-well). Cover and let rest 8 minutes before slicing.

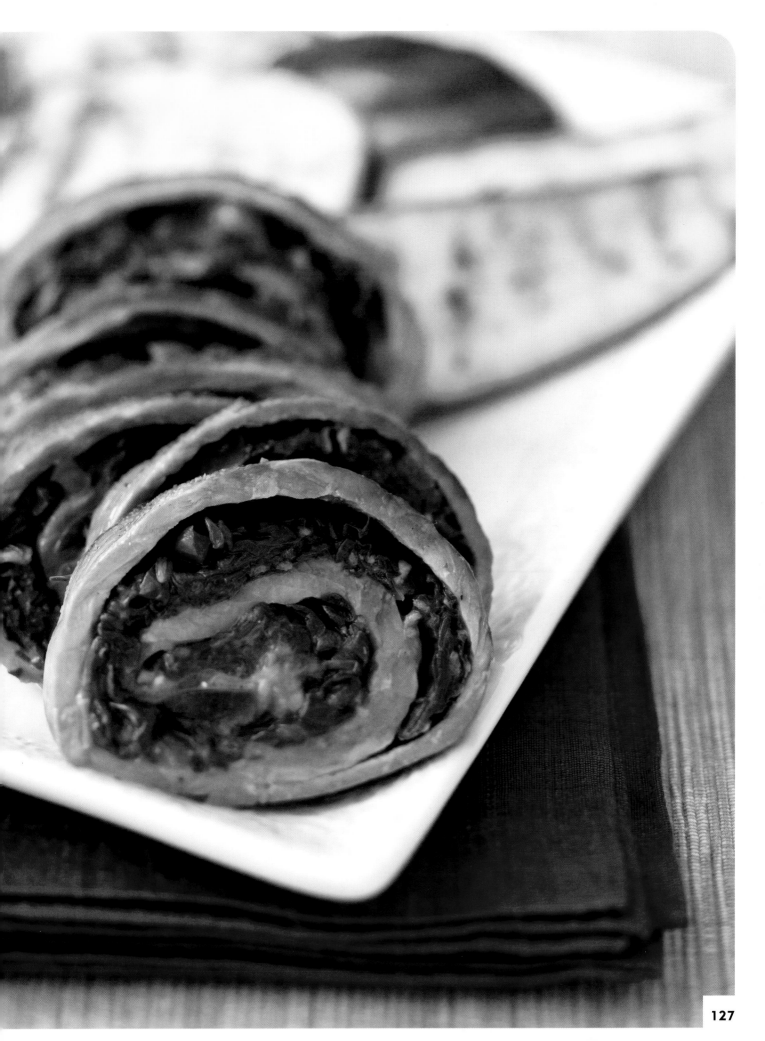

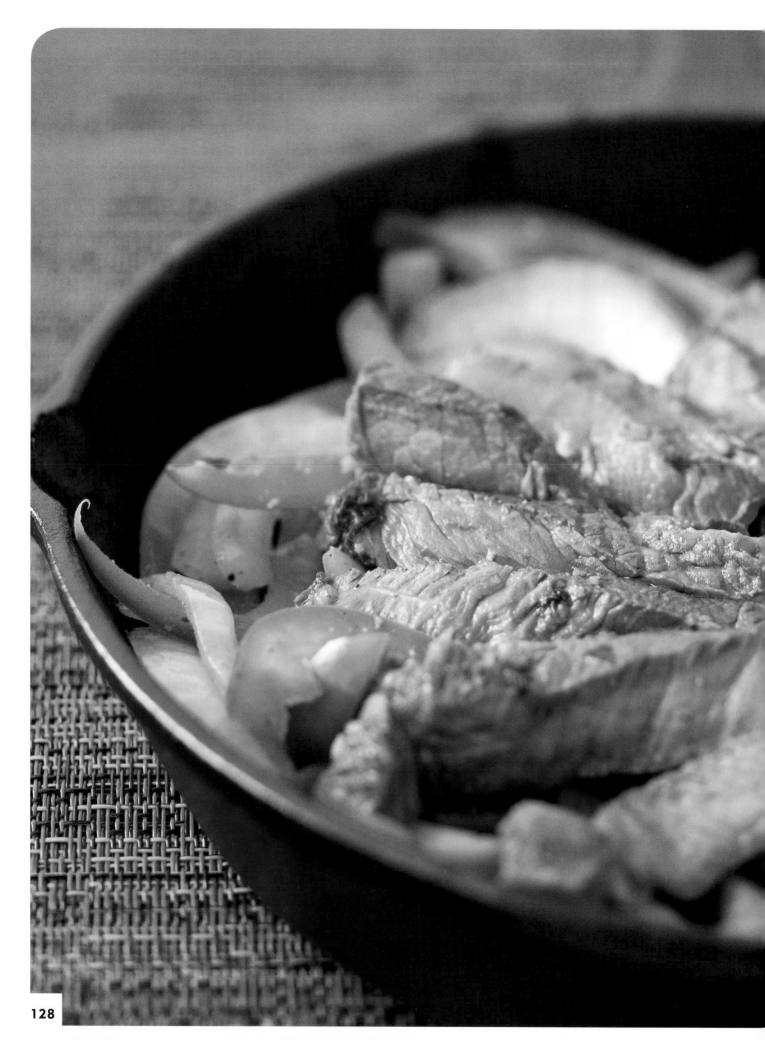

CALORIES	FAT	PROTEIN	CARBS	FIBER
380	14g	53g	8g	2g

SOUTHWESTERN PEPPER STEAK

"This southwestern recreation of the classic Asian pepper steak is a quick and easy way to prepare lower-fat top sirloin steaks with a whole lot of flavor."

YOU WILL NEED

4 cut top sirloin steaks (about 6 ounces each)

juice of 1 lime

1 tablespoon olive oil

2 cloves garlic, minced

3 tablespoons fresh chopped cilantro

½ teaspoon cumin

¼ teaspoon chili powder

⅛ teaspoon paprika

¼ teaspoon salt

⅛ teaspoon pepper

1 red bell pepper, sliced into strips

1 green bell pepper, sliced into strips

1 yellow onion, thinly sliced

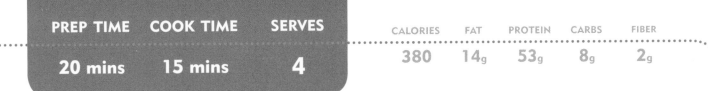

CHOOSE THIS!

Yellow Onions, especially the Vidalia variety, are wonderfully sweet onions that can add natural sugars to recipes that may otherwise require added refined sugar. In this recipe, sugar has been left out of the marinade for exactly that reason.

1 Place steaks in a food storage container and add lime juice, olive oil, garlic, cilantro, cumin, chili powder, paprika, salt, and pepper. Toss all to fully combine and coat steaks. Cover and refrigerate for at least 30 minutes.

2 Place a large skillet over medium-high heat and then drain about 1 tablespoon of the marinade that the steaks are in out of the food storage container into the skillet.

3 Add both red and green bell peppers and onions to the skillet and sauté until peppers are tender and onions are beginning to caramelize, about 6 minutes. Remove from pan and set aside.

4 Remove steaks from marinade and add to the hot skillet, searing for about 5 minutes on each side for medium doneness.

5 Add peppers and onions back into the pan and toss to reheat before serving the steaks smothered in them. You can also let the steaks rest 5 minutes and then slice before serving for an even nicer presentation.

LEAN MEATS

PINEAPPLE GLAZED HAM STEAKS

"These ham steaks are topped with whole pineapple rings and baked in a simple glaze made from only a few simple ingredients. I love the spice of ground cloves, but you can easily leave them out if they aren't for you."

YOU WILL NEED

1 ½ pounds ham steaks

8 canned pineapple rings, drained

2 tablespoons pineapple juice from can of rings

1 teaspoon Dijon mustard

1 tablespoon light brown sugar

⅛ teaspoon ground cloves

CHOOSE THIS!

Pineapple is extremely high in manganese, a trace mineral that can help your body build strong bones and connective tissue. Pineapple is also a great choice when you have colds, as it contains not only vitamin C but also bromelain, which can help suppress coughs.

1 Preheat oven to 375 degrees F. Line a sheet pan with aluminum foil.

2 Place ham steaks on the lined sheet pan and arrange pineapple rings over top.

3 In a small bowl, whisk together pineapple juice, Dijon mustard, brown sugar, and ground cloves. Drizzle over the pineapple-topped ham steaks.

4 Bake 10-15 minutes, just until ham steaks are warmed throughout and glaze is beginning to brown. Serve immediately.

VEGETABLE FILLED MEATLOAF

"Extra-lean ground beef has a real tendency to dry out, but this delicious meatloaf solves that problem by mixing high-moisture vegetables like zucchini and spinach right into the meat."

YOU WILL NEED

nonstick cooking spray

1 ½ pounds extra-lean ground beef

¼ cup diced yellow onion

¼ cup finely diced red bell pepper

⅔ cup grated zucchini

½ cup chopped spinach leaves

¼ cup Italian breadcrumbs

3 tablespoons grated Parmesan cheese

2 large egg whites, beaten

1 tablespoon parsley flakes

½ teaspoon garlic powder

1 teaspoon salt

¼ teaspoon pepper

1 Preheat oven to 350 degrees F. Spray a loaf pan with nonstick cooking spray.

2 In a large mixing bowl, combine all remaining ingredients, using your hands to thoroughly mix.

3 Press the meatloaf mixture into the greased loaf pan to eliminate any air bubbles.

4 Bake 60-70 minutes, or until internal temperature reaches 160 degrees F. Let cool 5 minutes before slicing. I like to serve this alongside organic ketchup made from natural sugar.

LEAN MEATS

CHOOSE THIS!

Zucchini is a great source of folate, potassium, and vitamin A. At only about 25 calories each and with the ability to quickly absorb flavors, zucchini make wonderful "fillers" to help you bulk up any dish with very little caloric or flavor impact.

HONEY GARLIC PORK TENDERLOIN

"Sweet and natural honey is the perfect thing to calm the up-front flavor of garlic in this quickly roasted pork tenderloin. It's truly rare that you can cook a roast this flavorful in under 25 minutes!"

YOU WILL NEED

1 pork tenderloin, about 1 ¼ pounds

1 tablespoon soy sauce

1 tablespoon minced garlic

2 teaspoons lemon juice

2 teaspoons olive oil

⅛ teaspoon pepper

2 tablespoons honey

CHOOSE THIS!

Garlic is arguably one of the most beneficial ingredients in this book. Known to lower blood pressure, lower cholesterol, and control blood sugar levels, garlic's most beneficial attribute might be its well-studied cancer fighting properties.

1 Place pork tenderloin in a food storage container with soy sauce, garlic, lemon juice, olive oil, and pepper, tossing all to coat. Cover and refrigerate for 30 minutes to marinate.

2 Preheat oven to 450 degrees F. Place marinated tenderloin on a sheet pan lined with aluminum foil and drizzle marinade over top.

3 Bake 15 minutes, reduce oven temperature to 350 degrees F., and then remove tenderloin from oven. Drizzle the entire surface of the pork with honey.

4 Bake an additional 10-12 minutes, or until a meat thermometer inserted into the thickest part registers 160 degrees F. Let rest under aluminum foil for 10 minutes before slicing to serve.

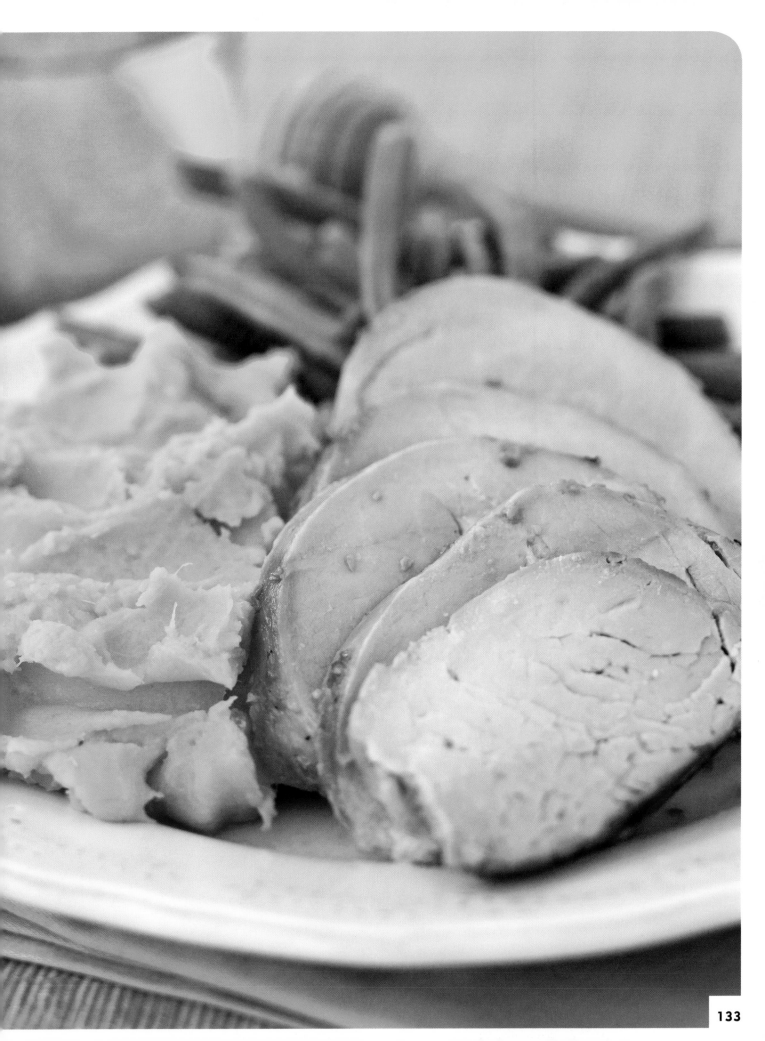

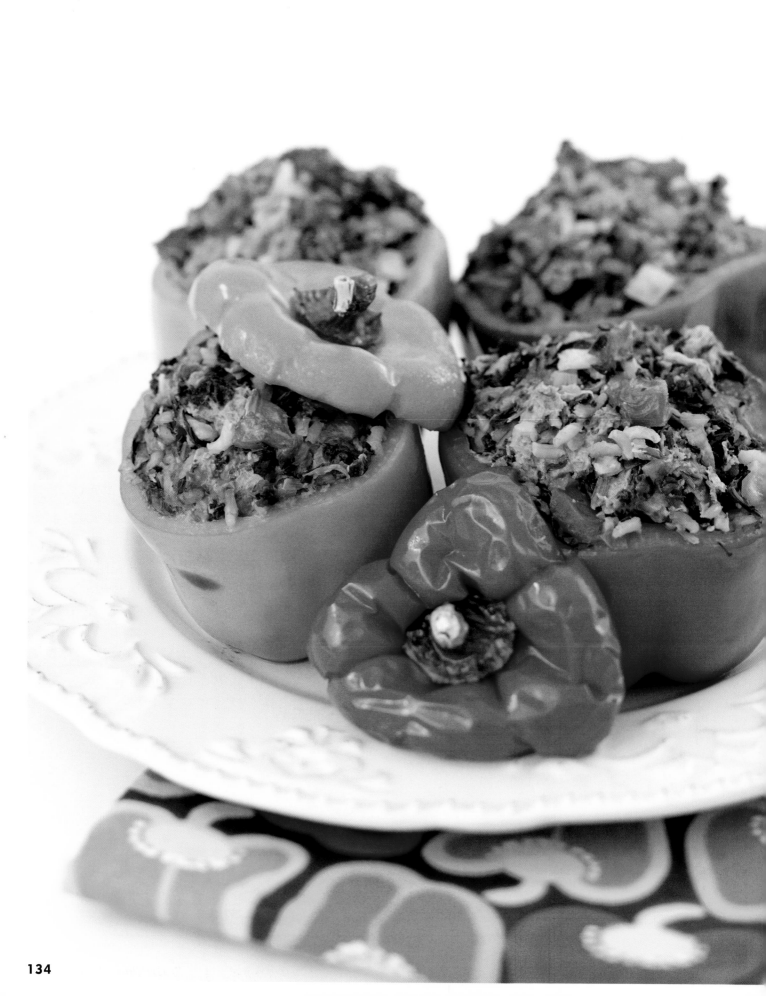

STUFFED PEPPERS

"Stuffed peppers are a perfect all-in-one meal with an even more perfect presentation. Choose the color of bell pepper based on your tastes; green are more savory, red are sweet, and yellow and orange are in the middle."

YOU WILL NEED

4 bell peppers of any color

nonstick cooking spray

¾ pound lean ground beef

1 cup cooked brown rice

10 ounces frozen chopped spinach, thawed and drained

1 tomato, diced

¼ cup diced yellow onion

2 tablespoons grated Parmesan cheese

2 teaspoons minced garlic

½ teaspoon dried oregano

½ teaspoon salt

¼ teaspoon pepper

1 Preheat oven to 350 degrees F. Cut tops off bell peppers and then scoop out and discard seeds. Spray the outside of peppers with nonstick cooking spray.

2 In a mixing bowl, combine all remaining ingredients to create the filling.

3 Fill each pepper with an equal amount of the filling and then place into a baking dish.

4 Bake 35-40 minutes, just until a meat thermometer inserted into the filling registers 160 degrees F. Serve immediately.

LEAN MEATS

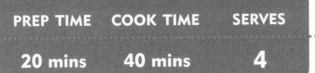

CHOOSE THIS!

Bell Peppers of all colors are loaded with vitamins A and C and several phytochemicals that can help protect cells from damage. Red bell peppers are my favorite because of their even higher nutrient content.

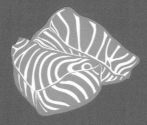

CATCH OF THE DAY

· ·

"Seafood can be one of the lowest-calorie and most delicious ways to get your fill of quality protein. It can also be one of your best sources for heart-healthy Omega-3 fatty acids."

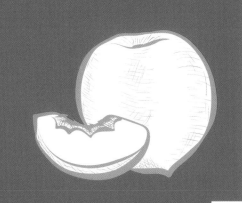

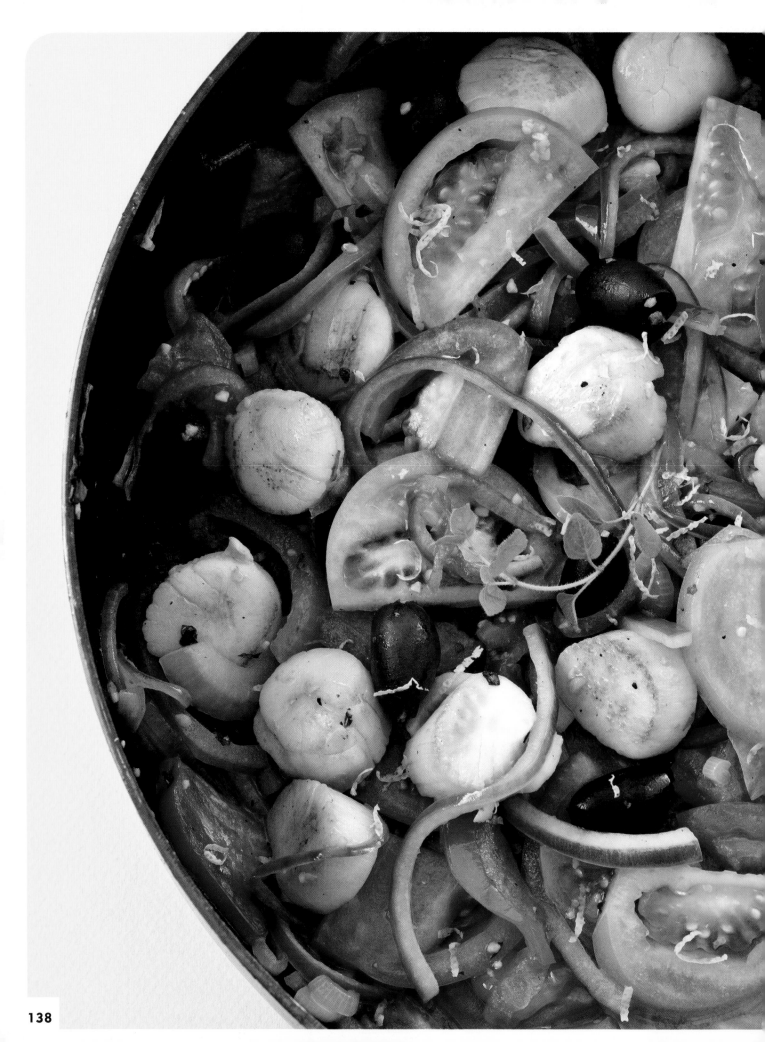

PREP TIME	COOK TIME	SERVES		CALORIES	FAT	PROTEIN	CARBS	FIBER
15 mins	15 mins	4		175	6g	20g	10.5g	2.5g

SEARED SCALLOPS WITH OLIVES AND TOMATOES

"This Mediterranean scallop dish with kalamata olives and two types of tomatoes is full of so many fresh flavors that it's hard to believe that it comes in at only 175 calories per serving!"

YOU WILL NEED

1 tablespoon olive oil

1 pound sea scallops

salt and pepper

1 red onion, thinly sliced

2 cloves garlic, minced

1 tomato, quartered and thinly sliced

1 green tomato, quartered and thinly sliced

⅓ cup pitted kalamata olives

¼ cup vegetable stock

1 tablespoon lemon juice

2 tablespoons fresh chopped oregano

¼ teaspoon lemon zest

1 Heat oil in a large skillet over medium-high heat.

2 Add scallops to the hot pan and season lightly with salt and pepper. Cook just until they begin to turn golden brown on both sides. Remove from pan and set aside.

3 Add onions to the pan and sauté until they begin to turn translucent.

4 Add garlic and cook 1 additional minute before adding all remaining ingredients and tossing to combine.

5 Return the scallops to the pan and sauté all together for 1-2 minutes, just until scallops are hot. Serve over rice, quinoa, couscous, or alongside your favorite sides.

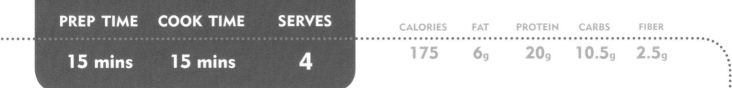

CHOOSE THIS!

Tomatoes are an excellent source of vitamins A, C, and K, but it's this mostly-savory fruit's lycopene content that truly sets it apart. Lycopene may reduce the risk for certain cancers and can even help maintain healthy blood pressure and strong bones.

CATCH OF THE DAY

PARMESAN CRUSTED TILAPIA

"Broiling white fish, especially tilapia, is not only delicious but also one of the fastest dinners you can make! In this recipe, tilapia is broiled with a delicious Parmesan cheese topping that cooks up golden brown and slightly crisp."

YOU WILL NEED

nonstick cooking spray

¼ cup grated Parmesan cheese

1 tablespoon olive oil

1 tablespoon lemon juice

2 tablespoons nonfat plain Greek yogurt

2 teaspoons breadcrumbs

⅛ teaspoon salt

⅛ teaspoon pepper

4 (6-ounce) tilapia fillets

CHOOSE THIS!

Tilapia, like most white fish, is low in fat, low in calories, and very rich in protein. Because tilapia are fast-growing and short-lived fish that eat a mostly vegetarian diet, they do not accumulate the mercury levels that some carnivorous fish do.

1 Preheat broiler to high. Line a sheet pan with aluminum foil and spray with nonstick cooking spray.

2 In a mixing bowl, combine Parmesan cheese, olive oil, lemon juice, yogurt, breadcrumbs, salt, and pepper to create the Parmesan crust.

3 Place tilapia fillets on the lined sheet pan and place about 5-6 inches under broiler. Broil for 6 minutes, flipping halfway through.

4 Spread Parmesan crust evenly over each of the tilapia fillets and then return to the broiler. Broil an additional 1-2 minutes, just until topping begins to brown and fish is flaky. Serve immediately.

HONEY MUSTARD SALMON

"The sweet honey and up-front flavor of coarse deli-style mustard perfectly complements the (good) fattiness of salmon in this simple seafood entrée made with minimal ingredients."

YOU WILL NEED

¼ cup coarse deli mustard

2 tablespoons honey

1 teaspoon minced garlic

2 teaspoons canola oil

1 ½ pounds salmon

nonstick cooking spray

CHOOSE THIS!

Salmon is a great source of essential omega-3 fatty acids, which are anti-inflammatory and play many important roles inside our bodies. These fatty acids are in fact essential, but our bodies do not create them on their own, so they must be present somewhere in our diet.

1 In a large mixing bowl, whisk together mustard, honey, garlic, and canola oil to create a marinade.

2 Cut salmon into 4 fillets and remove skin, if desired. (You can also ask the grocery store's seafood department to do this for you.)

3 Toss salmon in marinade, cover, and refrigerate for 30 minutes.

4 Preheat oven to 400 degrees F. Line a sheet pan with aluminum foil and then spray with nonstick cooking spray.

5 Place marinated salmon fillets on the lined sheet pan and then spread any remaining marinade over top.

6 Bake 12-16 minutes, or until salmon is opaque and easily flaked with a fork.

CATCH OF THE DAY

LEMON AND TARRAGON WHITEFISH

"This light entrée recipe for golden brown fish fillets in a butter, tarragon, and lemon sauce is made with white wine for an acidity that perfectly complements the fish."

YOU WILL NEED

2 teaspoons olive oil

1 ½ pounds whitefish fillets (tilapia, cod, halibut, etc.)

salt and pepper

⅓ cup dry white wine

1 tablespoon lemon juice

1 teaspoon minced garlic

2 teaspoons chopped fresh tarragon

¼ teaspoon finely grated lemon zest

1 tablespoon light butter

⅛ teaspoon salt

⅛ teaspoon pepper

CHOOSE THIS!

Lemons, like most citrus fruit, are abundant with vitamin C. It is commonly used in household cleaning products as its citric acid is a potent disinfectant. These same disinfectant qualities can actually cleanse your stomach and boost your immunity.

1 Heat oil in a large skillet over medium to medium–high heat.

2 Pat fish dry with paper towels and season lightly with salt and pepper.

3 Add seasoned fish to the hot pan and sear until golden brown, about 2 minutes on each side. The fish is done when it easily flakes with a fork. Remove from pan and cover with aluminum foil to keep warm.

4 Whisk white wine, lemon juice, and minced garlic into the pan to start the sauce. Let simmer 2 minutes before adding tarragon and lemon zest. Let simmer 1 additional minute.

5 Remove sauce from heat and stir in butter, salt, and pepper. Toss fish in sauce before serving drizzled with additional sauce.

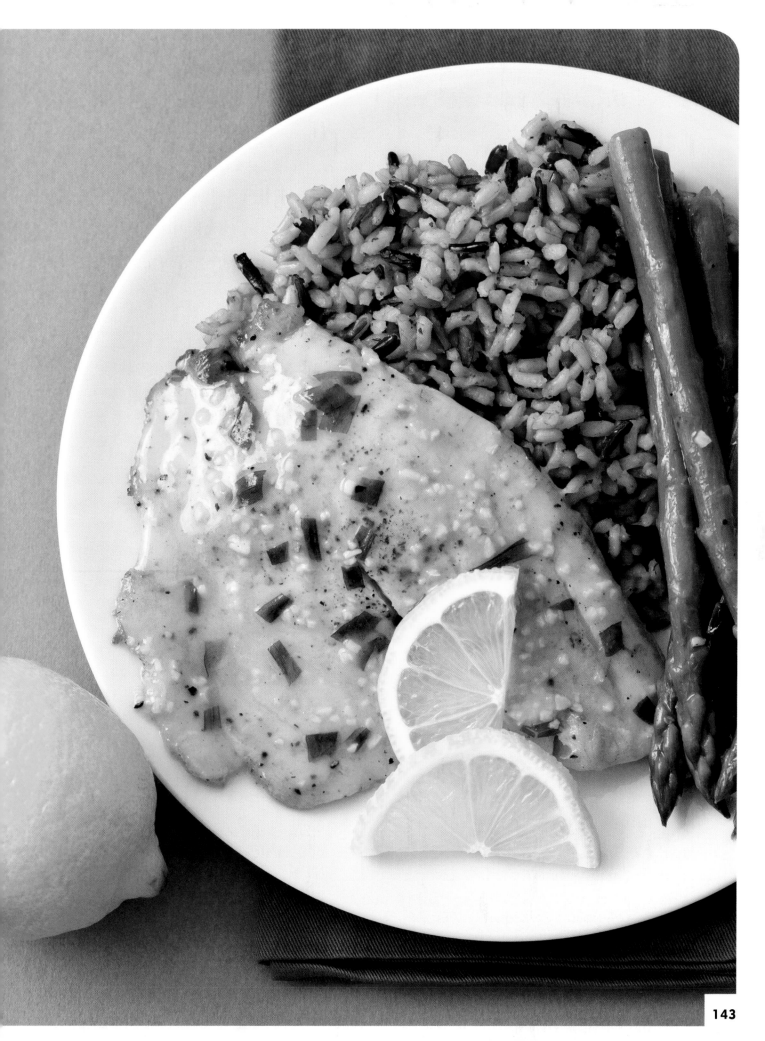

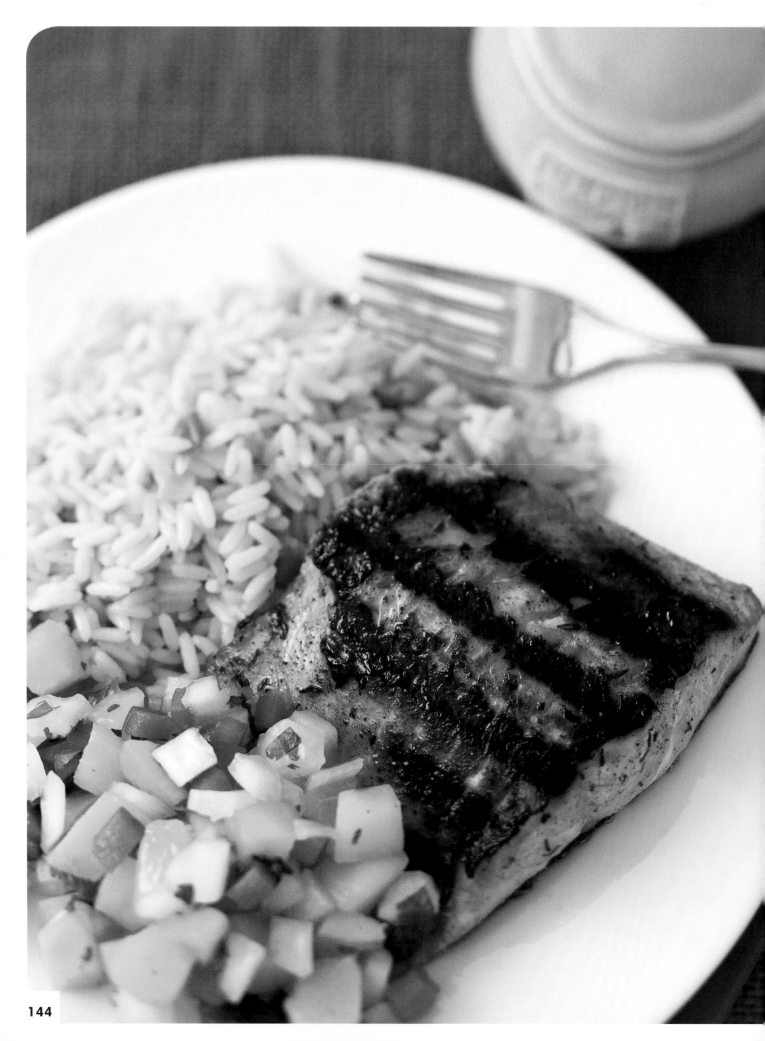

GRILLED SALMON WITH PEACH SALSA

"This salmon is marinated in tropical spices, grilled, and then served alongside a savory and sweet peach salsa for the perfect combination of fresh flavors."

YOU WILL NEED

PEACH SALSA

2 peaches, diced
¼ cup finely diced yellow onion
¼ cup finely diced red bell pepper
¼ cup fresh cilantro, chopped
1 tablespoon honey
2 teaspoons lemon juice
⅛ teaspoon salt

GRILLED SALMON

1 ½ pounds salmon
1 tablespoon olive oil
2 teaspoons honey
1 teaspoon lemon juice
¼ teaspoon dry thyme
¼ teaspoon ground allspice
¼ teaspoon salt
⅛ teaspoon pepper

1 In a mixing bowl, combine all Peach Salsa ingredients, tossing well. Cover and refrigerate until ready to serve.

2 Cut salmon into 4 fillets and remove skin, if desired. (You can also ask the grocery store's seafood department to do this for you.)

3 In a large mixing bowl, whisk together all remaining Grilled Salmon ingredients to create a marinade. Toss salmon in marinade, cover, and refrigerate for 30 minutes.

4 Lightly oil a grill, indoor grill, or grill pan and set to high heat.

5 Grill marinated salmon 5-7 minutes on each side, cooking until the fish is easily flaked with a fork. Serve topped with a generous portion of the Peach Salsa.

CATCH OF THE DAY

CHOOSE THIS!

Peaches are a juicy and succulent source of beta-carotene, which not only gives them their peachy color but also helps protect our eyes, heart, and other organs.

PREP TIME	COOK TIME	SERVES		CALORIES	FAT	PROTEIN	CARBS	FIBER
20 mins	20 mins	4		474	7g	41g	64g	9g

WHOLE WHEAT TUNA NOODLE DINNER

"This all-in-one tuna noodle dinner makes 4 huge and nutritionally-balanced portions that are sure to satisfy the entire family."

YOU WILL NEED

8 ounces whole wheat rotini or elbow noodles

1 tablespoon light butter

8 ounces baby bella mushrooms, sliced

⅓ cup finely diced red onion

2 cups fresh snap peas

1 teaspoon minced garlic

1 (12-ounce) can fat-free evaporated milk

½ cup chicken broth

¼ cup all-purpose flour

½ teaspoon dry thyme

¼ teaspoon lemon pepper

12 ounces (canned or pouched) chunk light tuna, drained

⅓ cup shredded Parmesan cheese

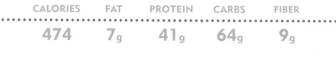

CHOOSE THIS!

Tuna is not only a wonderfully lean, high-quality protein, but it is also an amazing source of omega-3 fatty acids, potassium, selenium, and vitamin B12. While mercury levels have been of discussion in recent years, the chunk light tuna in this recipe has been proven to be the safest.

1 Bring a large pot of lightly-salted water to a boil. Add pasta and cook according to package directions. Drain well.

2 Meanwhile, heat butter in a large skillet over medium-high heat. Add mushrooms and onion, and cook until mushrooms begin to cook down, about 4 minutes.

3 Add snap peas and minced garlic to the pan and sauté 2 additional minutes.

4 Whisk together evaporated milk, chicken broth, and flour, and then pour into the pan. Add thyme and lemon pepper and bring all up to a simmer. Let simmer 2 minutes, until a thick sauce is created.

5 Fold in drained tuna, Parmesan cheese, and cooked pasta, and heat just 1 minute to warm the tuna. Serve immediately.

PREP TIME	COOK TIME	SERVES		CALORIES	FAT	PROTEIN	CARBS	FIBER
10 mins	12 mins	4		360	14g	51g	3.5g	0g

GRILLED TERIYAKI TUNA STEAKS

"These thick and hearty tuna steaks are marinated in an Asian marinade that caramelizes extremely well on the grill, making for something not only delicious but also extremely presentable. Serve with brown rice and green vegetables for the perfect meal."

YOU WILL NEED

3 tablespoons low-sodium soy sauce

1 tablespoon rice wine vinegar

1 tablespoon sesame oil

1 tablespoon light brown sugar

2 green onions, thinly sliced

⅛ teaspoon ground ginger

4 (6-ounce) tuna steaks

CHOOSE THIS!

Low-Sodium Soy Sauce is a great way to enjoy Asian flavors with about 50% less salt content than the regular version. Because sodium attracts and holds water, it can actually increase blood volume, putting a strain on your heart if you consume more than your kidneys can excrete.

1 In a wide dish, combine soy sauce, rice wine vinegar, sesame oil, brown sugar, green onions, and ground ginger to create a marinade.

2 Place tuna steaks in marinade and toss to coat. Cover and refrigerate for at least 30 minutes to marinate.

3 Lightly oil a grill, indoor grill, or grill pan and set to high heat.

4 Grill marinated tuna steaks 4-6 minutes on each side, cooking until the fish is easily flaked with a fork. Serve immediately.

PREP TIME	COOK TIME	SERVES		CALORIES	FAT	PROTEIN	CARBS	FIBER
25 mins	10 mins	4		430	13.5g	29g	48.5g	5g

SHRIMP WITH CILANTRO-LIME RICE

"This sautéed shrimp dish with bell peppers, diced tomatoes, and green onions is served over cilantro and lime infused brown rice for a fully fresh meal with great southwestern flavors."

YOU WILL NEED

3 tablespoons olive oil

1 cup uncooked brown rice

¼ cup lime juice

2 cups water

2 tablespoons fresh chopped cilantro

3 cloves garlic, minced

1 red bell pepper, diced

1 pound shrimp, peeled and deveined

2 tomatoes, diced

6 green onions, thinly sliced

¼ teaspoon salt

⅛ teaspoon pepper

CHOOSE THIS!

Brown Rice is a whole grain that has a mild nutty flavor. It is slightly chewier but far more nutritious and fiber-rich than the white rice it substitutes. While white rice does have some of the same nutrients as brown rice, these nutrients are usually lower-quality synthetic versions that are added after processing, called "fortifying".

1 In a 3 quart saucepan, heat 1 tablespoon of the olive oil over high heat. Add the brown rice and lime juice, and cook for 1 minute before adding the water.

2 Bring rice mixture up to a boil, cover, and then reduce heat to low. Let cook until all water is absorbed, about 25-30 minutes. Stir in cilantro and season with salt and pepper to taste.

3 Meanwhile, heat the remaining 2 tablespoons of olive oil in a large skillet over medium heat. Add the garlic and bell pepper to the skillet and sauté for 4 minutes, or until bell pepper is nearly tender.

4 Add shrimp to the skillet and cook until all shrimp have turned pink, about 4 minutes.

5 Add diced tomatoes, green onions, salt, and pepper to the shrimp and sauté just until tomatoes are heated through and are beginning to release their juices. Remove from heat.

6 Serve shrimp and vegetable mixture over the cilantro-lime rice.

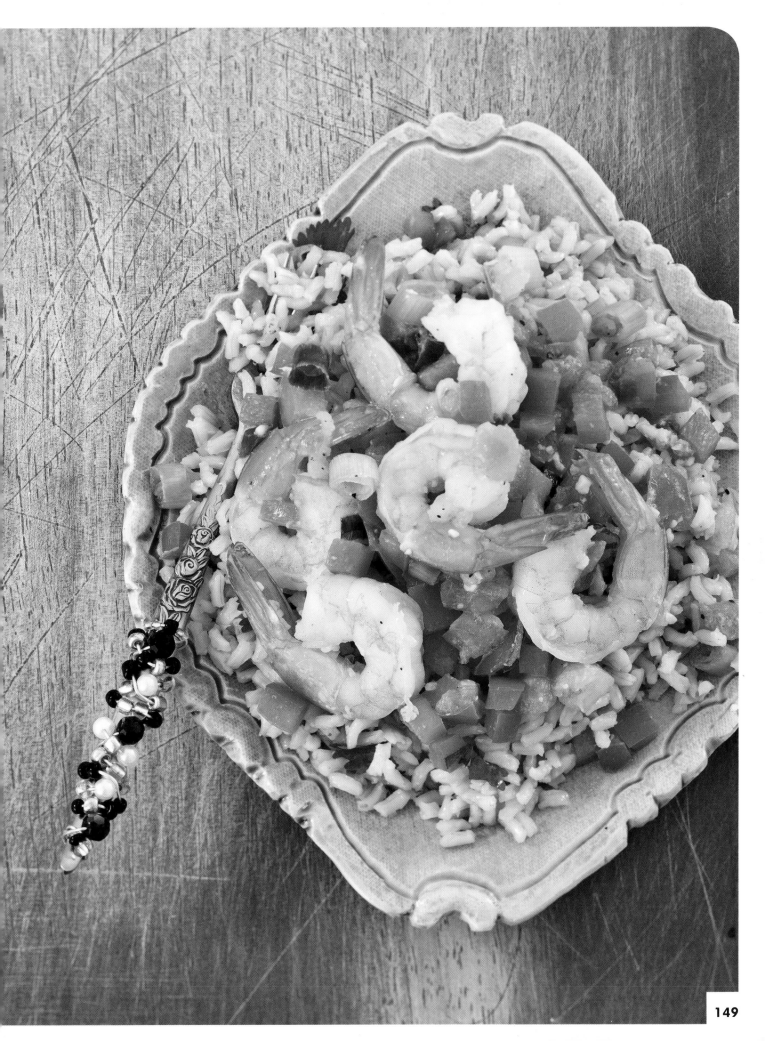

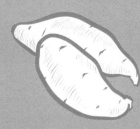

CHOOSING SIDES

"Side dishes and vegetables quite literally complete the meal! Try to aim for at least 3 different colors of vegetables a day to maximize your vitamin and mineral intake."

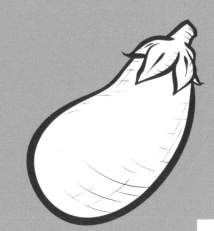

PREP TIME	COOK TIME	SERVES		CALORIES	FAT	PROTEIN	CARBS	FIBER
15 mins	15 mins	4		185	12g	11g	11g	2g

SOY GLAZED BROCCOLI AND TOFU

"Robust soy sauce combines with sweet rice wine vinegar to make this dish of sautéed broccoli and seared tofu a taste sensation."

YOU WILL NEED

1 (14-ounce) package firm tofu

½ cup low-sodium soy sauce

¼ cup rice wine vinegar

2 teaspoons sesame oil

2 cloves garlic, minced

1 teaspoon ground ginger

2 tablespoons olive oil

1 (12-ounce) bag fresh broccoli florets

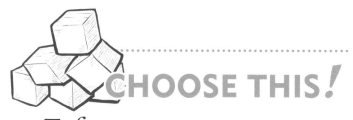

CHOOSE THIS!

Tofu is a great vegetarian source of protein and a great vegan source of calcium. In fact, this side dish could easily be served over brown rice as a well balanced vegan entrée.

1 Drain tofu and slice into ½-inch wide by 1-inch long pieces. Place on a clean kitchen towel and let drain of excess moisture for 30 minutes.

2 In a mixing bowl, combine soy sauce, rice wine vinegar, sesame oil, minced garlic, and ground ginger.

3 Heat olive oil in a large skillet over medium heat. Add drained tofu pieces to the skillet and let cook without stirring until golden brown. Flip and cook on each side until all sides are this color.

4 Add the soy sauce mixture and broccoli florets to the skillet and toss until tofu and broccoli are fully saturated with the sauce.

5 Cover and cook until broccoli is tender, about 5 minutes. Serve immediately.

PREP TIME	COOK TIME	SERVES		CALORIES	FAT	PROTEIN	CARBS	FIBER
20 mins	none	4		85	1g	3g	18g	3.5g

FENNEL SLAW

"Fennel bulbs are a truly wonderful vegetable with a very mild licorice-like flavor and a crunch that is very similar to celery. It's the absolutely perfect crunch for a creamy slaw recipe like this one."

YOU WILL NEED

⅔ cup fat-free sour cream

1 tablespoon white wine vinegar

2 teaspoons lemon juice

1 teaspoon light brown sugar

⅛ teaspoon dried thyme

1 bulb fennel, peeled, cored, and thinly sliced

1 granny smith apple, julienned

1 cup thinly sliced celery

¼ yellow onion, thinly sliced

1 In a mixing bowl, whisk together sour cream, white wine vinegar, lemon juice, brown sugar, and thyme to create a dressing.

2 For best results: use a mandolin to thinly slice and julienne the vegetables for this slaw.

3 Place vegetables in a large serving bowl and pour dressing over top. Toss all to combine.

4 Cover and refrigerate at least 30 minutes to let the flavors combine before serving.

CHOOSE THIS!

Fennel is actually an herb that is closely related to dill. This recipe calls for the bulb of the fennel, which has a texture that is very similar to celery and is very high in fiber and potassium.

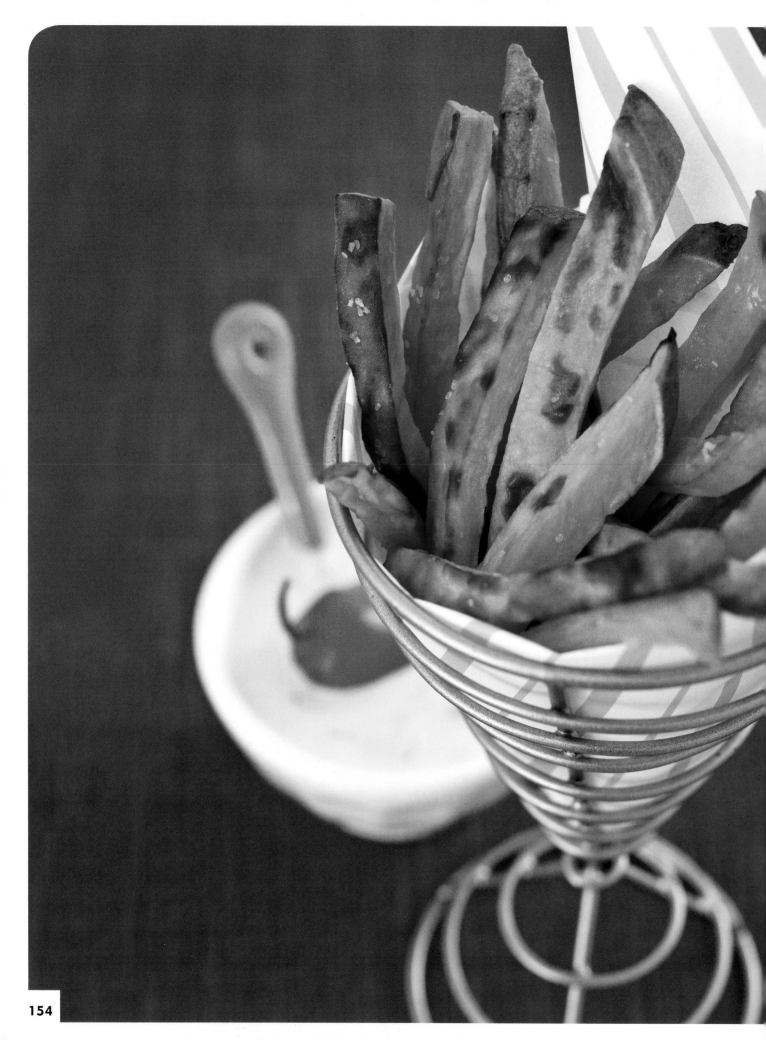

SWEET POTATO FRIES WITH CHIPOTLE SAUCE

"These baked sweet potato fries are a delicious and much more nutritious alternative to deep fried white potatoes! I like to serve them with this spicy chipotle chili dipping sauce to cut the sweetness of the potatoes."

YOU WILL NEED

3 sweet potatoes, washed

2 tablespoons olive oil

salt

1 cup fat-free sour cream

2 tablespoons canned chipotle chilies in adobo sauce, seeds removed and diced

2 tablespoons lime juice

¼ cup fresh cilantro, chopped

CHOOSE THIS!

Sweet Potatoes are an excellent source of beta-carotene, which not only gives them their red color, but also helps protect our eyes, heart, and other organs. Eating sweet potatoes with the skin on will help you get the most of their rich nutrient and fiber content.

1 Preheat oven to 350 degrees F. Cut potatoes into long, thin sticks.

2 Toss the cut potatoes in olive oil and then spread out across a large sheet pan. Sprinkle with a generous amount of salt.

3 Bake 40-45 minutes, flipping halfway through, until potatoes are brown and crispy on the outside.

4 Meanwhile, prepare the Chipotle Sauce by combining all remaining ingredients. Add salt to taste, cover, and refrigerate until ready to serve.

5 Serve the baked sweet potato fries immediately with the Chipotle Sauce for dipping.

CHOOSING SIDES

SNAPPY PEAS

"Snap peas are some of the quickest and easiest fresh vegetables to prepare. It is a common misconception that they require the time-consuming removal of their stems before cooking. Here, I've paired the sweet pea pods with olive oil and lemon for a simple and delicious side dish."

YOU WILL NEED

1 pound snap peas

1 tablespoon olive oil

1 teaspoon lemon juice

1 ½ teaspoons lemon zest

¼ teaspoon salt

⅛ teaspoon pepper

1 Place snap peas in a pot of boiling water and boil 2 minutes, just until tender but still snappy.

2 Drain snap peas well and then return to the stove over medium heat. Add all remaining ingredients and toss to fully coat.

3 Cook just 1 minute before removing from heat and serving immediately.

CHOOSE THIS!

Snap Peas, also known as sugar snap peas, contain 4 grams of heart-healthy fiber and only 65 calories per cup. Though they are great cooked, their sweet taste and satisfying crunch also make them a healthier choice for dipping into savory dips in place of potato chips.

PREP TIME	COOK TIME	SERVES		CALORIES	FAT	PROTEIN	CARBS	FIBER
15 mins	15 mins	4		75	3g	2g	10.5g	4.5g

SAUTÉED EGGPLANT WITH CARAMELIZED ONIONS

"I find eggplant to be one of the most underused vegetables around. Their ability to absorb even the subtlest of flavors while also adding their own mild and unique flavor makes dishes like this more complex in taste than the simple ingredients would have you believe."

YOU WILL NEED

1 tablespoon light butter

1 large yellow onion, thinly sliced

1 eggplant, cubed

2 cloves garlic, minced

¼ teaspoon salt

⅛ teaspoon pepper

¼ cup vegetable broth

1 tablespoon chopped parsley

1 Place butter in a large nonstick skillet over medium-high heat.

2 Once butter has melted, add onions and sauté 5 minutes, or until onions turn a light brown.

3 Add eggplant, garlic, salt, and pepper to the pan and sauté 3 minutes before adding vegetable broth.

4 Continue cooking, stirring constantly, for 5-8 minutes, or until eggplant is tender. Stir in parsley and serve immediately.

CHOOSE THIS!

Eggplant is a great choice for sautés or stir-fries because of its uncanny ability to absorb flavors. Eggplant is high in fiber, phytonutrients, and potassium that (along with the fruit's natural water content) can help keep you hydrated.

PREP TIME	COOK TIME	SERVES		CALORIES	FAT	PROTEIN	CARBS	FIBER
20 mins	6 mins	24		95	2g	3.5g	18.5g	6.5g

EASY GRILLED ITALIAN VEGETABLES

"Grilled vegetables are one of my go-to side dishes that I prepare in some kind of form at least once a week. Using an electric indoor grill allows me to cook the rest of my meal on the stove as these are grilling."

YOU WILL NEED

1 large eggplant

2 zucchini

2 red bell peppers

1 red onion

1 cup fat-free Italian salad dressing

salt and pepper

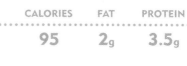

CHOOSE THIS!

Zucchini is a great source of folate, potassium, and vitamin A. Zucchini's ability to easily absorb flavors is definitely on display in this recipe, as they take on the smoky charred flavors of the grill extremely well.

1 Cut ends from eggplant and slice into ½-inch thick discs. Cut ends from zucchini and slice lengthwise into ½-inch thick strips. Cut red bell pepper away from the core in 4 big pieces by slicing down on each of its four sides. Peel and slice onion into ½-inch thick slices.

2 Place sliced vegetables on a large sheet pan and pour salad dressing over top all. Let sit 30 minutes to marinate.

3 Lightly oil a grill, indoor grill, or grill pan and set to high heat.

4 Grill vegetables 2-3 minutes on each side, until well-marked by the grill and tender to your grilling tongs. Watch vegetables carefully, as they may finish cooking 1-2 minutes apart from each other depending on thickness and hot spots on the grill. Transfer vegetables onto a serving platter as they finish cooking.

5 Lightly season with salt and pepper and serve immediately.

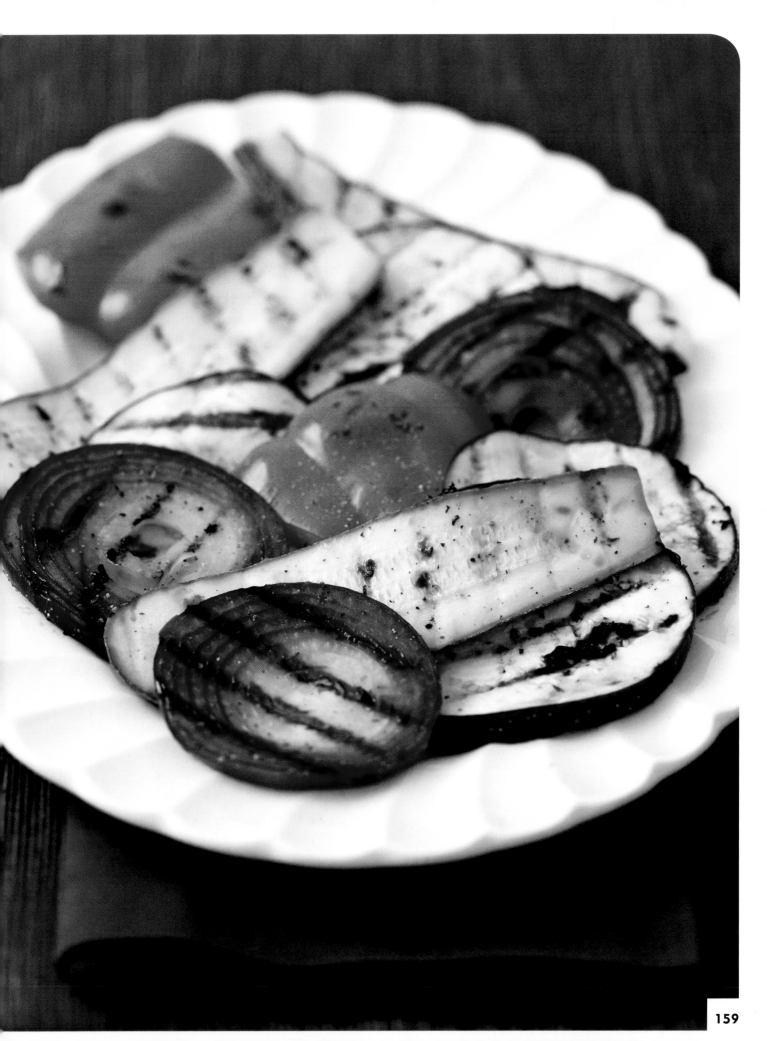

BROCCOLI GRATIN

"This baked broccoli dish is topped with a crunchy topping made from Parmesan cheese and ground almonds that toast up nice and aromatic as the gratin bakes."

YOU WILL NEED

nonstick cooking spray

1 large bunch broccoli, separated into florets

½ cup low-fat milk

2 large egg whites

¼ teaspoon salt

⅛ teaspoon pepper

⅛ teaspoon garlic powder

¼ cup almonds

½ cup grated Parmesan cheese

CHOOSE THIS!

Broccoli is arguably one of the healthiest foods on the planet. Not only does broccoli contain more fiber than whole wheat bread but it also has more vitamin C than an orange and just as much calcium as a glass of milk!

1 Preheat oven to 400 degrees F. Spray a 2 quart baking dish with nonstick cooking spray.

2 Place broccoli florets in a pot of boiling water and boil 5 minutes, just until tender but still crisp.

3 Drain broccoli well and then place in the greased baking dish.

4 In a mixing bowl, whisk together milk, egg whites, salt, pepper, and garlic powder. Pour mixture over broccoli in baking dish and then toss to fully coat.

5 Place almonds and Parmesan cheese into a food processor and pulse until almonds are finely ground and dispersed throughout the cheese. Sprinkle this mixture over top the coated broccoli in the baking dish.

6 Bake 10-12 minutes, just until almond and Parmesan mixture begins to brown. Let cool 5 minutes before serving.

PREP TIME	COOK TIME	SERVES		CALORIES	FAT	PROTEIN	CARBS	FIBER
20 mins	1+ hour	6		195	3g	9.5g	33g	4g

LOW-FAT SCALLOPED POTATOES

"These scalloped potatoes bake up in a thick, creamy, and Parmesan cheesy sauce while still managing to come in at only 3 grams of fat per serving. While white potatoes get bad press, take notice that, thanks to potatoes, this recipe has 4 grams of healthy fiber."

YOU WILL NEED

nonstick cooking spray

4 potatoes, thinly sliced

5 green onions, thinly sliced

1 (12-ounce) can fat-free evaporated milk

1 tablespoon light butter, melted

⅓ cup grated Parmesan cheese

3 tablespoons all-purpose flour

¼ teaspoon salt

⅛ teaspoon pepper

⅛ teaspoon garlic powder

1 Preheat oven to 375 degrees F. Spray a 2 quart baking dish with nonstick cooking spray.

2 Place sliced potatoes in the baking dish, sprinkling the sliced green onions between layers of the potatoes.

3 In a mixing bowl, whisk together all remaining ingredients and pour over top of the potatoes in the baking dish. Shake dish to help the liquid settle.

4 Cover with aluminum foil and bake 50 minutes. Uncover and bake an additional 20 minutes, or until potatoes are fork tender. Let cool at least 5 minutes to set before serving.

CHOOSE THIS!

Low-Fat Evaporated Milk

gives these potatoes a thick and creamy sauce with only about ¼ of the calories of the more traditional heavy cream. Be careful not to purchase sweetened condensed milk (a sugar overload!) by accident; it is definitely NOT the same thing.

CHOOSING SIDES

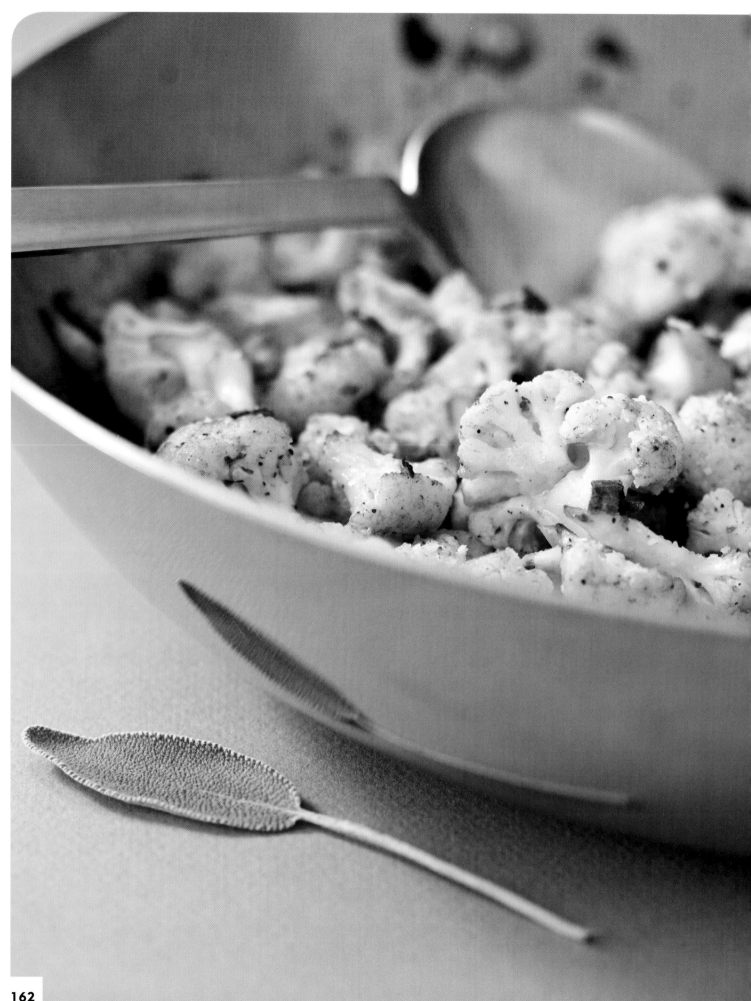

GOLDEN CAULIFLOWER WITH SAGE

"This recipe is a play on an Italian way of preparing ravioli; only instead, it is made into a side dish by substituting cauliflower in place of the ravioli. The cauliflower, sautéed in (light) butter and sage, actually caramelizes and takes on a wonderful, almost nutty flavor."

YOU WILL NEED

1 head cauliflower

1 tablespoon light butter

1 tablespoon olive oil

¼ teaspoon salt

⅛ teaspoon pepper

¼ cup water

6 sage leaves, chopped

2 tablespoons grated Parmesan cheese

⅛ teaspoon garlic powder

CHOOSE THIS!

Cauliflower, like its close relative broccoli, is one of the healthiest foods on the planet. While it is high in fiber, vitamin C, antioxidants, and calcium, I think my favorite thing about cauliflower is how well it can absorb flavors like the sage in this dish. You can also make this dish with a mixture of regular and purple cauliflower for a really beautiful presentation.

1 Cut cauliflower into tiny florets, each about the size of a quarter, discarding the large stem.

2 Heat butter and oil in a large skillet over medium-high heat.

3 Once the pan is hot, add cauliflower florets, salt, and pepper and toss once to coat florets in oil.

4 Sauté, stirring occasionally until cauliflower is well browned all the way around.

5 Stir water and sage into the pan and continue sautéing until water has almost completely evaporated.

6 Stir in Parmesan cheese and garlic powder and remove pan from heat. Serve immediately.

CHOOSING SIDES

PREP TIME	COOK TIME	SERVES		CALORIES	FAT	PROTEIN	CARBS	FIBER
15 mins	10 mins	6		110	6.5g	1g	13g	2g

GLAZED CARROT MEDALLIONS

"These sweet and buttery carrot medallions are caramelized in a light brown sugar glaze that makes them irresistible to kids and, well, just about everyone. I'm not a fan of overcooked, soft carrots, so this recipe also retains just the right amount of the carrot's natural crunch."

YOU WILL NEED

2 tablespoons butter

1 tablespoon canola oil

4 cups peeled and sliced carrots, about ¼ inch thick

¼ cup light brown sugar

¼ teaspoon salt

⅓ cup water

1 Place butter and oil in a large nonstick skillet over medium-high heat.

2 Once butter has melted, add carrots and sauté 3 minutes before stirring in brown sugar and salt. Cook just until sugar has melted.

3 Pour water into the pan and sauté until almost all of the water has reduced into a thick, caramel-like sauce that thoroughly coats the carrots. If carrots are not as tender as you would like, add additional water, repeating this step again. Serve hot.

CHOOSE THIS!

Carrots are most known for their amazingly high beta-carotene content. This beta-carotene not only gives them their bright orange color but also helps protect our eyes, heart, and other organs.

PREP TIME	COOK TIME	SERVES		CALORIES	FAT	PROTEIN	CARBS	FIBER
10 mins	50 mins	4		105	3g	1g	21g	2g

HONEY ROASTED BUTTERNUT SQUASH

"I roast this butternut squash in the skin until the pulp is as smooth and creamy as mashed sweet potatoes. Drizzling with a little honey when roasting enhances the squash's natural sweetness and highlights its great, nutty flavor."

YOU WILL NEED

1 butternut squash

1 tablespoon butter, melted

¼ teaspoon pumpkin pie spice

¼ teaspoon salt

2 tablespoons honey

CHOOSE THIS!

Butternut Squash, once cooked, has a wonderfully creamy texture without any fat or cholesterol. It is also a very good source of fiber, vitamin C, and beta-carotene, which can help protect your eyes, heart, and other organs.

1 Preheat oven to 375 degrees F. Line a baking dish with aluminum foil.

2 Cut butternut squash in half and remove seeds by scraping with a heavy spoon. Place halves in the lined baking dish, cut-side up.

3 In a small bowl, combine melted butter, pumpkin pie spice, and salt, and drizzle over the butternut squash in the baking dish.

4 Bake squash 20 minutes before removing and drizzling with the honey. Return to the oven and bake an additional 20-30 minutes, or until squash is tender. Spoon out of the rind to serve.

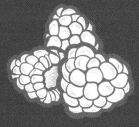

SMOOTHIE TIME!

· ·

"I have a sweet tooth and a home-made smoothie can be one of the best ways to satisfy that need for sweets while still having something nutritious and energizing."

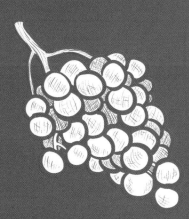

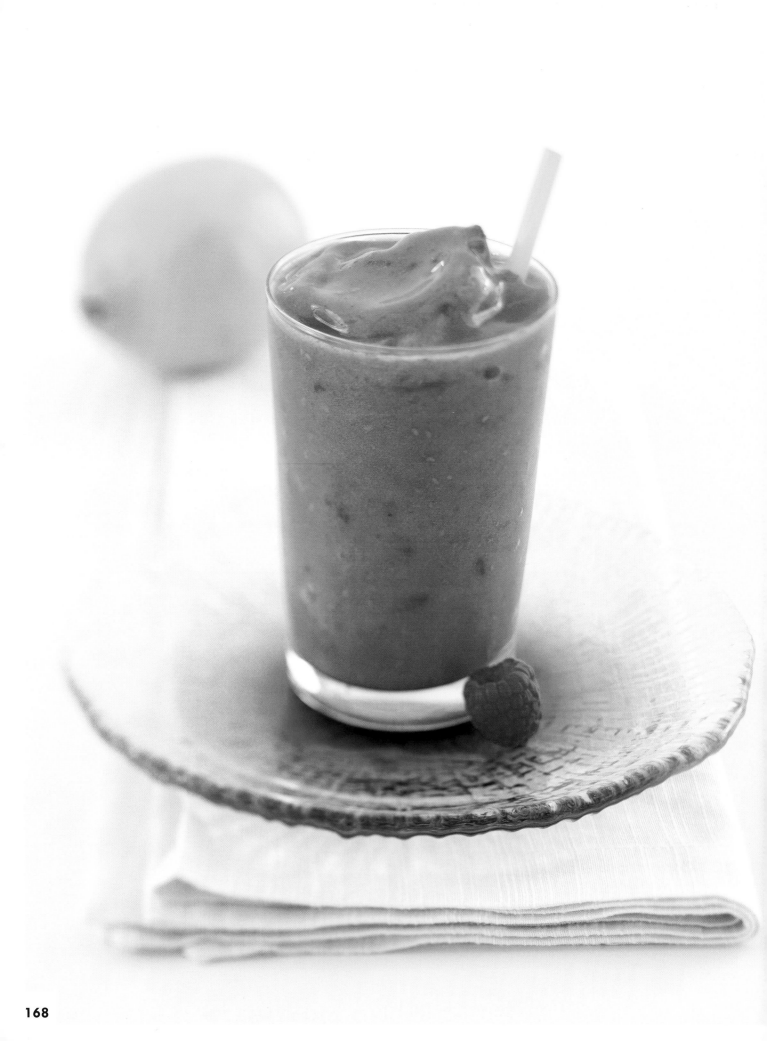

RASPBERRY LEMON PUCKER SMOOTHIE

"The taste of this tart smoothie reminds me of those rocket pops (with the red, white, and blue layers) that I'd get from the ice cream man growing up. The natural fruitiness of the raspberries offsets the tartness of the lemon."

SMOOTHIE TIME!

YOU WILL NEED

½ cup frozen raspberries

½ cup lemon sherbert (may use sorbet)

¾ cup diet lemonade

1 Place all ingredients into a blender.

2 Pulse a few times to roughly chop the frozen raspberries before blending until drink is entirely smooth, about 1 minute. Serve immediately.

CHOOSE THIS!

Raspberries are a very good source of manganese, a trace mineral that helps raise your metabolism. When combined with their decent amount of natural fiber, manganese makes raspberries an amazing fat-burning food. Like most berries, raspberries are also a great source of antioxidants, including vitamin C.

PUMPKIN PIE SMOOTHIE

"This smoothie has all of the taste of pumpkin pie along with all of the protein and fiber of a satisfying, meal-replacing smoothie. When else can you get away with eating pumpkin pie for breakfast?"

YOU WILL NEED

½ cup canned pumpkin

1 (6-ounce) container nonfat plain Greek yogurt (may use regular yogurt)

1 tablespoon light agave nectar (may use honey)

¾ cup almond milk

½ teaspoon pumpkin pie spice

½ teaspoon vanilla extract

5 ice cubes

1 Place all ingredients into a blender, adding ice first or last (depending on your blender) to keep it closest to the blades.

2 Pulse a few times to roughly chop the ice before blending until drink is entirely smooth, about 1 minute. Serve immediately.

3 You can also split this smoothie into 2-3 parfait glasses, top them with small dollops of a low-fat whipped topping, and serve for dessert.

CHOOSE THIS!

Almond Milk is a wonderfully rich and creamy substitute for whole milk or half and half. Some brands of almond milk (such as *Almond Breeze*) can even have as little as 40 calories per cup, which is less than ⅓ of the calories of whole milk! Not just a great alternative to higher-fat dairy, it is also great for those with soy allergies who are prevented from consuming soy milk.

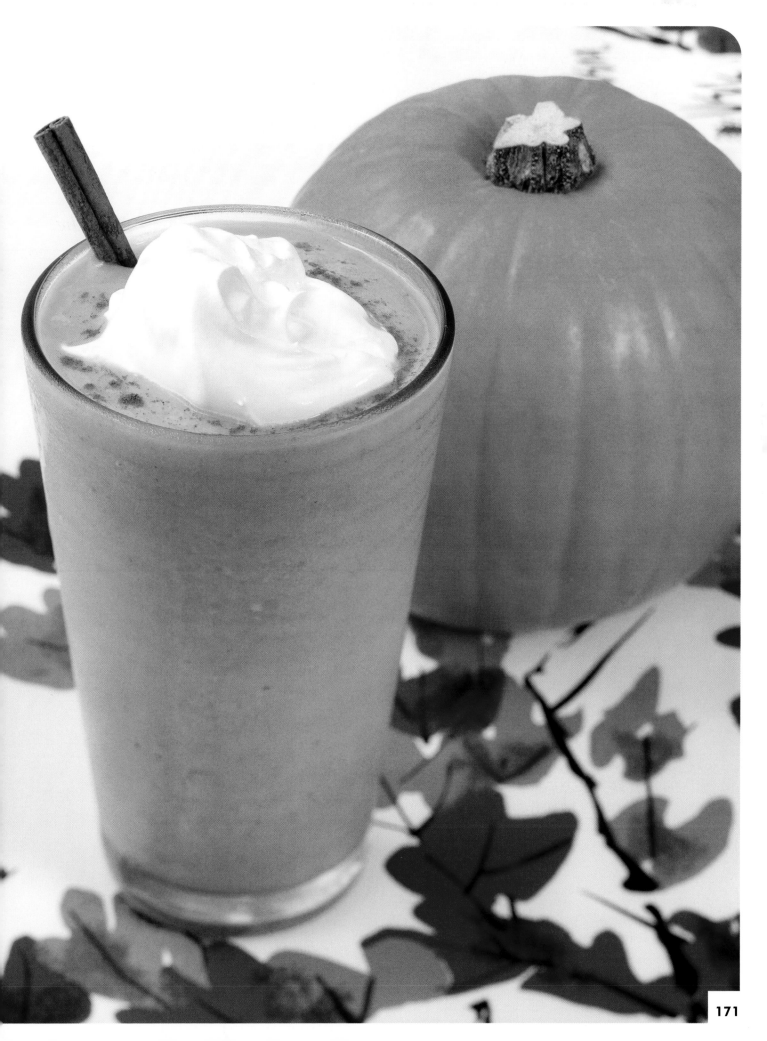

PREP TIME	COOK TIME	SERVES		CALORIES	FAT	PROTEIN	CARBS	FIBER
5 mins	none	1		195	0.5g	24g	26g	3g

POPEYE SMOOTHIE

"Although this smoothie's color can easily give away the fact that it is loaded with a boost of healthy spinach leaves, I promise you that the frozen peaches and pineapples that are blended in as well make this a delicious treat that truly tastes nothing like it looks!"

YOU WILL NEED

½ cup frozen peach slices

½ cup frozen pineapple chunks

1 (6-ounce) container nonfat plain Greek yogurt (may use regular yogurt)

1 cup fresh spinach leaves

1 cup diet sweetened iced tea (diet green tea beverages are best!)

1 Place all ingredients into a blender.

2 Pulse a few times to roughly chop the frozen fruit before blending until drink is entirely smooth, about 1 minute. Serve immediately.

CHOOSE THIS!

Spinach is loaded with vitamins, minerals, and antioxidants, which truly makes this smoothie a knockout. When you combine the spinach with the peaches and pineapple, this recipe gives you 3 of your 5-9 recommended fruit and vegetable servings for the day.

"CHOCOLATE COVERED BANANA" MALT

"This recipe is great for a quick on-the-go breakfast, post-workout snack, or even a delicious malted milkshake-like dessert."

YOU WILL NEED

1 banana

1 cup light soy milk

1 tablespoon malt powder

2 tablespoons sugar-free chocolate instant pudding mix

1 Peel and slice banana, placing the slices on a parchment paper-lined plate. Freeze until slices are frozen solid.

2 Place frozen banana slices and all remaining ingredients into a blender.

3 Pulse a few times to roughly chop the bananas before blending until drink is entirely smooth, about 1 minute. Serve immediately.

CHOOSE THIS!

Bananas are best known for being extremely high in potassium, which is an electrolyte that can be depleted during a vigorous workout. Without an adequate supply of potassium, you are susceptible to painful leg cramps, so be sure to enjoy this smoothie as a delicious post-workout replenisher.

SMOOTHIE TIME!

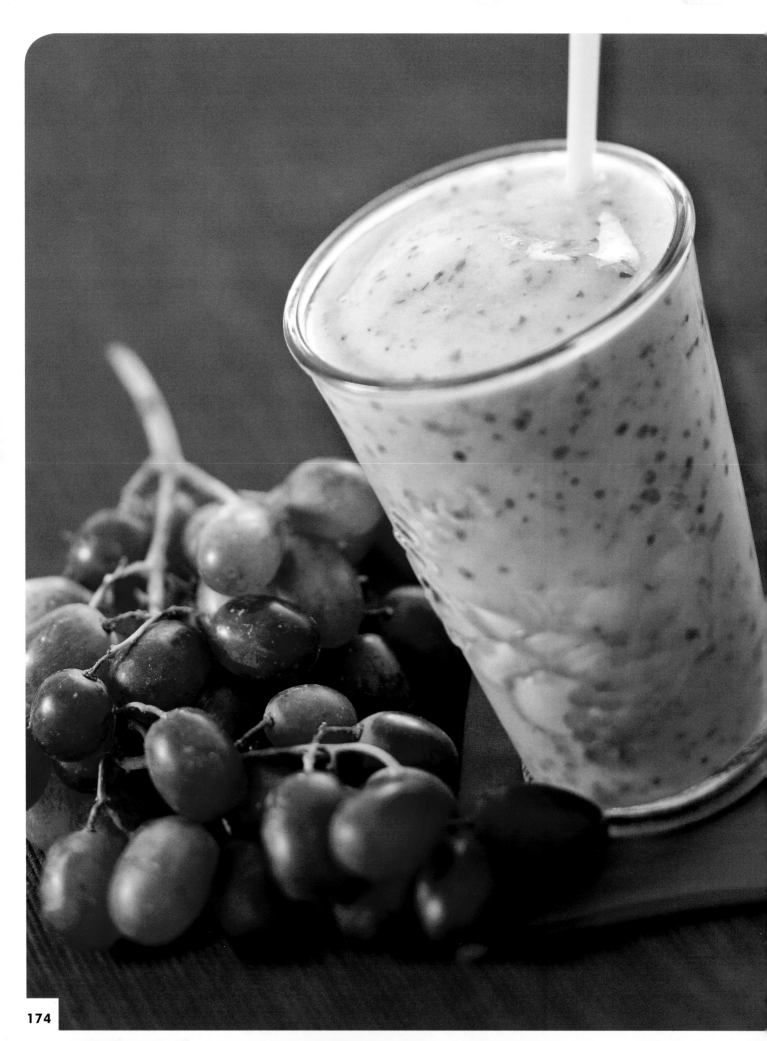

GROOVY GRAPE SMOOTHIE

"Freezing fresh grapes and adding them to a smoothie instead of ice cubes makes for an incredibly smooth texture that is also rich with nutrients. In this recipe, I've added grape juice to make the grape flavor more pronounced and a little bit of banana and strawberry yogurt to make it 'Groovy'."

YOU WILL NEED

1 cup red seedless grapes

⅓ banana, peeled and chopped

½ cup nonfat strawberry yogurt

½ cup grape juice

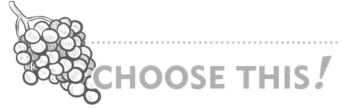

CHOOSE THIS!

Grapes and grape juice are wonderful sources of potent flavonoids that may even be responsible for many of the well-known health benefits of drinking a glass of red wine a day. Flavonoids are plant compounds that act as antioxidants in the body and may reduce the risk of heart disease.

1 Freeze grapes for at least 2 hours, or until frozen solid.

2 Place frozen grapes and all remaining ingredients into a blender.

3 Pulse a few times to roughly chop the frozen grapes before blending until drink is entirely smooth, about 1 minute. Serve immediately.

SMOOTHIE TIME!

PREP TIME	COOK TIME	SERVES		CALORIES	FAT	PROTEIN	CARBS	FIBER
5 mins	none	1		85	1.5g	3.5g	11g	0g

FROZEN COFFEE SHOPACCINOS

"Skip the lines, the cost, and a whole lot of fat by preparing creamy frozen coffee drinks at home!"

YOU WILL NEED

½ cup double-strength coffee (may substitute 2 teaspoons instant coffee dissolved in ½ cup water)

¼ cup fat-free half and half

2 tablespoons bulk sugar substitute (or 3 packets)

½ cup ice

¼ teaspoon vanilla extract

1 Cool coffee completely before preparing.

2 Place coffee and all remaining ingredients into a blender.

3 Pulse a few times to roughly chop the ice before blending until drink is entirely smooth, about 1 minute. Serve immediately.

CHOOSE THIS!

Fat-Free Dairy, such as the fat-free half and half used in this drink can save you a ton of calories over their full-fat alternatives while still giving you that creamy coffee bliss you crave. Often, a coffee shop smoothie like this one contains regular half and half or even high-fat heavy cream to get that creaminess. My recipe has less than 2g of fat, but preparing the same recipe with heavy cream would bring that up to 11g!

PREP TIME	COOK TIME	SERVES	CALORIES	FAT	PROTEIN	CARBS	FIBER
10 mins	none	1	180	1g	6.5g	41g	5g

KIWI-DEW SMOOTHIE

"Don't let the green color of this smoothie deter you from enjoying its refreshing and somewhat tropical flavor. For something even more cool and refreshing, try throwing in a few slices of ice cold cucumber!"

YOU WILL NEED

½ cup chopped honeydew melon (may use cantaloupe)

2 kiwis, peeled and chopped

½ cup nonfat vanilla yogurt

½ cup bottled diet green tea

5 ice cubes

1 Place all ingredients into a blender.

2 Pulse a few times to roughly chop the fruit before blending until drink is entirely smooth, about 1 minute. Serve immediately.

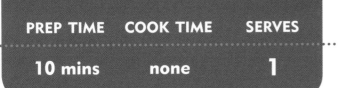

CHOOSE THIS!

Kiwis are absolutely bursting with immune system boosting vitamin C. In fact, you can get more than 100% of your daily recommended value of vitamin C in just one 50 calorie kiwi! Kiwis are also a good source of dietary fiber, potassium, magnesium, manganese, and vitamin E.

PREP TIME	COOK TIME	SERVES		CALORIES	FAT	PROTEIN	CARBS	FIBER
5 mins	none	1		145	2g	2g	29g	4.5g

STRAWBERRIES AND CREAM SMOOTHIE

"This delicious dessert smoothie is thick, creamy, and the closest thing you can get to a milkshake in under 150 calories! In fact, I think that using real strawberries gives this drink the edge over the artificially flavored milkshakes (that are hardly ever even made from actual ice cream) served in most places these days."

YOU WILL NEED

1 ¼ cups frozen strawberries

¾ cup almond milk

2 tablespoons fat-free half and half (may use additional almond milk)

1 tablespoon light brown sugar

¼ teaspoon vanilla extract

1 Place all ingredients into a blender.

2 Pulse a few times to roughly chop the frozen strawberries before blending until drink is entirely smooth, about 1 minute. Serve immediately.

CHOOSE THIS!

Strawberries are filled with anthocyanins that not only provide their flush red color but also serve as potent antioxidants that have been shown to help protect the body's cells from free radical damage. This makes these delicious little berries a heart protecting, anti-inflammatory, and possibly even cancer preventing fruit all rolled into one.

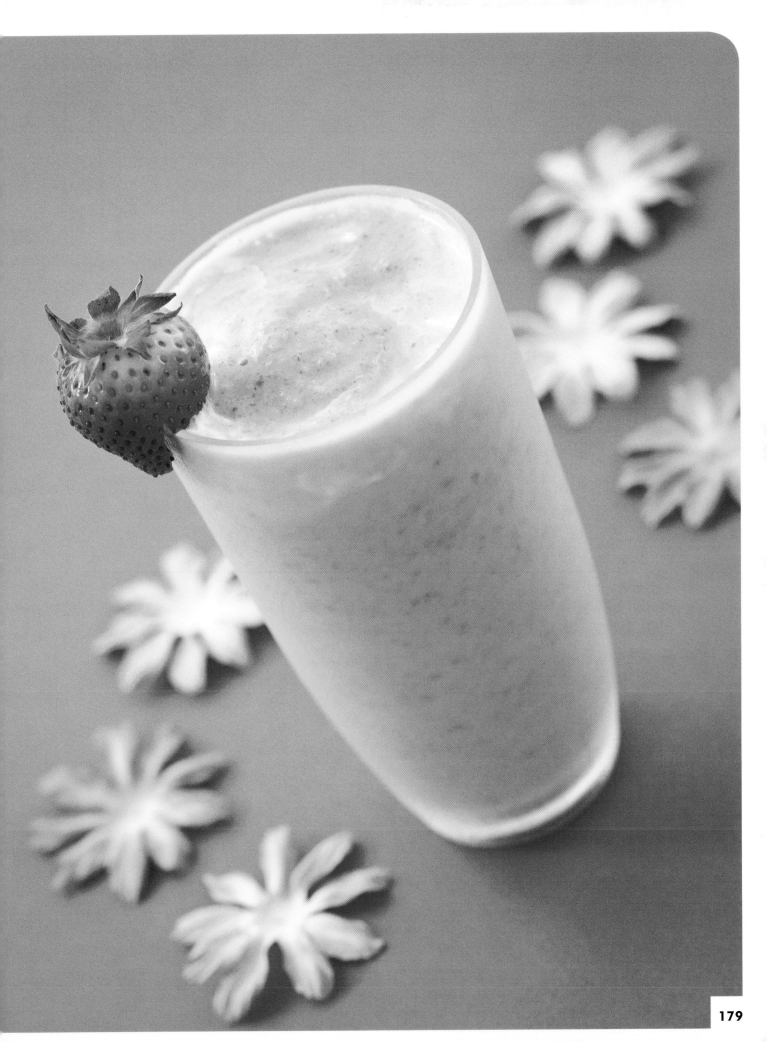

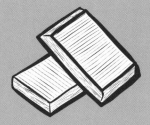

THE SWEET STUFF

"There is no need to deny yourself dessert. Choosing healthier, fresher desserts with reasonable portions will allow you to have your cake and eat it without regrets!"

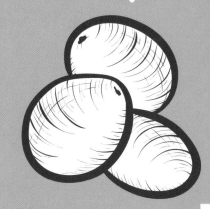

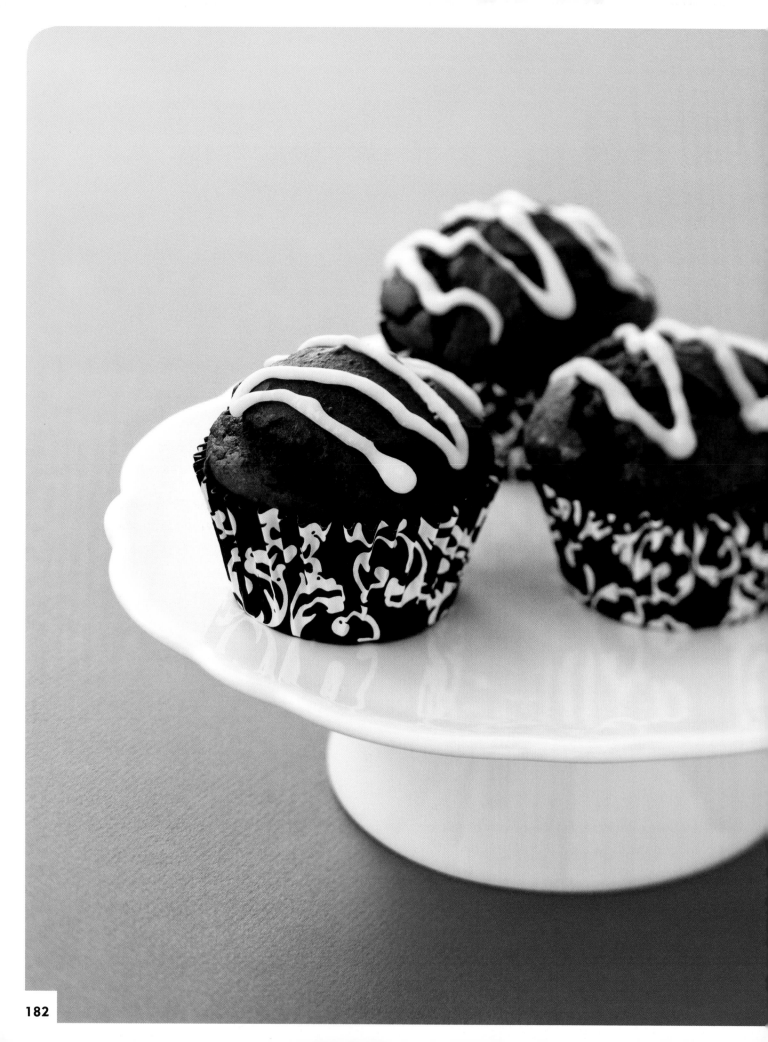

PREP TIME	COOK TIME	SERVES		CALORIES	FAT	PROTEIN	CARBS	FIBER
15 mins	24 mins	24		120	3.5g	2g	22.5g	1g

YES YOU CAN CUPCAKES

"These chocolate cupcakes are an amazing feat at only 120 calories each. What's even more amazing is that they actually start with ordinary cake mix and still make it in with that number of calories. The secret is substituting canned pumpkin (which is masked by the rich chocolate) for the oil and egg yolks you would normally use.

YOU WILL NEED

1 (18.5-ounce) box dark chocolate cake mix

1 (16-ounce) can pumpkin

2 large egg whites

½ cup water

1 full cup confectioners sugar

¼ teaspoon vanilla extract

1 ½ tablespoons water

CHOOSE THIS!

Pumpkin is extremely high in anti-oxidants and beta-carotene, which can help regenerate cells in the body. This effect makes it a great "age reversing" food. Its smooth consistency helps keep these cupcakes moist without any added oil.

1 Preheat oven to 350 degrees F. Line cupcake pans with 24 cupcake liners.

2 In an electric mixer, beat chocolate cake mix, pumpkin, egg whites, and ½ cup water for 2 minutes to create a smooth batter.

3 Pour batter into the prepared cupcake liners, filling them about ⅔ of the way full.

4 Bake 20-24 minutes, or until a toothpick inserted into the center of a cupcake comes out mostly clean.

5 In a microwave-safe bowl, combine confectioners sugar, vanilla extract, and 1 ½ tablespoons water to create the icing. Microwave 30 seconds, just until icing is fully combined and smooth.

6 Drizzle icing over all cupcakes and let cool completely to set before serving.

ALMOND KISSED MACAROONS

"These sweet and flaky coconut macaroons are topped with whole almonds and drizzled with dark chocolate for a truly decadent end to any meal."

YOU WILL NEED

nonstick cooking spray

1 ½ cups sweetened dried coconut flakes

¼ cup sugar

2 large egg whites, beaten

1 teaspoon vanilla extract

16 whole almonds

3 ounces dark chocolate

CHOOSE THIS!

Almonds are regarded as one of the healthiest nuts (though they are technically seeds) with an amazing ability to raise good HDL cholesterol as it lowers bad LDL cholesterol. This "super food" is also high in fiber, magnesium, potassium, and a host of other important vitamins and minerals.

1 Preheat oven to 350 degrees F. Spray a large baking sheet with nonstick cooking spray.

2 In a large mixing bowl, fold together coconut, sugar, egg whites, and vanilla extract until well combined.

3 Use a tablespoon to scoop rounded spoonfuls of the mixture onto the greased baking sheet, spacing them about 2 inches apart.

4 Place a whole almond into the center of each mound of dough.

5 Bake 12-15 minutes, or until macaroons are lightly browned.

6 As the cookies are cooling, place chocolate in a microwave-safe dish and microwave on high for 1-2 minutes, stirring every 30 seconds, until entirely melted.

7 Drizzle melted chocolate over the almonds in the center of the baked macaroons. Let cool completely before serving.

PREP TIME	COOK TIME	SERVES		CALORIES	FAT	PROTEIN	CARBS	FIBER
10 mins	15 mins	8		90	2g	1g	19g	2g

ROASTED FIGS WITH MINT CHOCOLATE DRIZZLE

"Fresh figs are an extremely underused ingredient that are available in almost every grocery store (near the fresh berries). This simple dessert with sweet baked figs drizzled in a chocolate mint sauce is great for getting accustomed to these high-fiber fruits."

YOU WILL NEED

nonstick cooking spray

8 figs

2 tablespoons light brown sugar

2 ounces dark chocolate, chopped

½ teaspoon fresh chopped mint

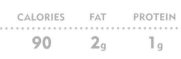

CHOOSE THIS!

Fresh Mint has been used medicinally for all manners of things for centuries. Rich in vitamins A and C—as well as essential minerals like manganese, copper, iron, and potassium—its best attribute might be its ability to fight off bad breath when eating a dessert like this one after a meal with garlic or onions!

1 Preheat oven to 350 degrees F. Spray a baking dish with nonstick cooking spray.

2 Cut figs in half lengthwise and place in the greased baking dish cut-side up. Sprinkle brown sugar over top all.

3 Bake figs for 10-15 minutes, just until figs begin to soften and sugar begins to caramelize. Transfer two fig halves to each serving plate.

4 Place chocolate in a microwave-safe bowl and microwave in 15-second intervals, stirring in between, until chocolate has completely melted. Stir in fresh mint.

5 Drizzle melted chocolate over the fig halves on each serving plate and serve immediately. Figs are entirely edible, including the skin.

STRAWBERRY FILLED MERINGUE "NESTS"

"These desserts are conveniently self-portioned and are an elegant and fresh way to re-invent the humble meringue cookie. This also makes a great base recipe for "nests" to fill with your favorite fruits or ingredients!"

YOU WILL NEED

4 large egg whites, room temperature

¼ teaspoon cream of tartar

¾ cup sugar

1 cup strawberries, freshly sliced

¼ cup sugar

4 large dollops Cool Whip Light

CHOOSE THIS!

Egg Whites are pure protein without the calories, fat, or cholesterol of whole eggs. In most recipes, including baked goods, 2 egg whites can easily substitute 1 whole egg with very little impact on the final dish.

1 Preheat oven to 250 degrees F. In a large mixing bowl, beat egg whites with an electric mixer until foamy. Add the cream of tartar and continue beating until soft peaks form.

2 Slowly add the first measure of sugar (¾ cup) to the egg whites as you continue beating. Beat until sugar is entirely incorporated and stiff peaks are formed.

3 On a parchment paper-lined sheet pan, make 6 equal piles of the meringue. Use the back of a spoon to press an indent into the top of each pile, creating the look of a "nest".

4 Bake for 1 hour before turning the oven off with the meringue nests still inside. Let nests sit in the warm oven for at least 3 hours, or until dry to the touch.

5 In a small mixing bowl, combine strawberries and the second measure of sugar (¼ cup). Let sit, stirring occasionally, until strawberries have released their juice and created a sauce with the sugar.

6 Serve baked nests filled with an equal portion of strawberries and topped with a large dollop of Cool Whip.

PREP TIME	COOK TIME	SERVES		CALORIES	FAT	PROTEIN	CARBS	FIBER
15 mins	5 mins	16		135	7.5g	2.5g	18.5g	1.5g

PISTACHIO AND CRANBERRY CHOCOLATE BARK

"Dark chocolate is far healthier than the milk variety, but when I am in the mood for something a little more interesting, I make a delicious dark chocolate bark like this one with toasted pistachios and dried cranberries."

YOU WILL NEED

1 cup shelled pistachios, chopped

8 ounces dark chocolate, chopped

1 cup dried sweetened cranberries

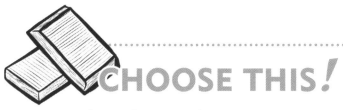

CHOOSE THIS!

Dark Chocolate is rich in heart healthy plant compounds called flavonoids. These flavonoids are present in all chocolate, but milk chocolate is so watered down with milk fat and sugar that the amount becomes insignificant. Look for 70% or darker chocolate to maximize your benefits.

1 For best flavor, toast pistachios on a sheet pan for 4-5 minutes in a 350 degree F. oven before preparing. Toast just until they smell aromatic.

2 Line a sheet pan with parchment paper.

3 Place chopped chocolate in a metal or tempered-glass mixing bowl and place over a pot of simmering water to create a double boiler.

4 Stir the chocolate constantly, until entirely melted.

5 Pour melted chocolate onto the parchment paper-lined sheet pan and spread until about ⅓ inch thick.

6 Sprinkle toasted pistachios and sweetened cranberries over the entire surface of the melted chocolate. Use a rubber spatula to press all down into the chocolate.

7 Let cool completely, until firm. Break apart and serve.

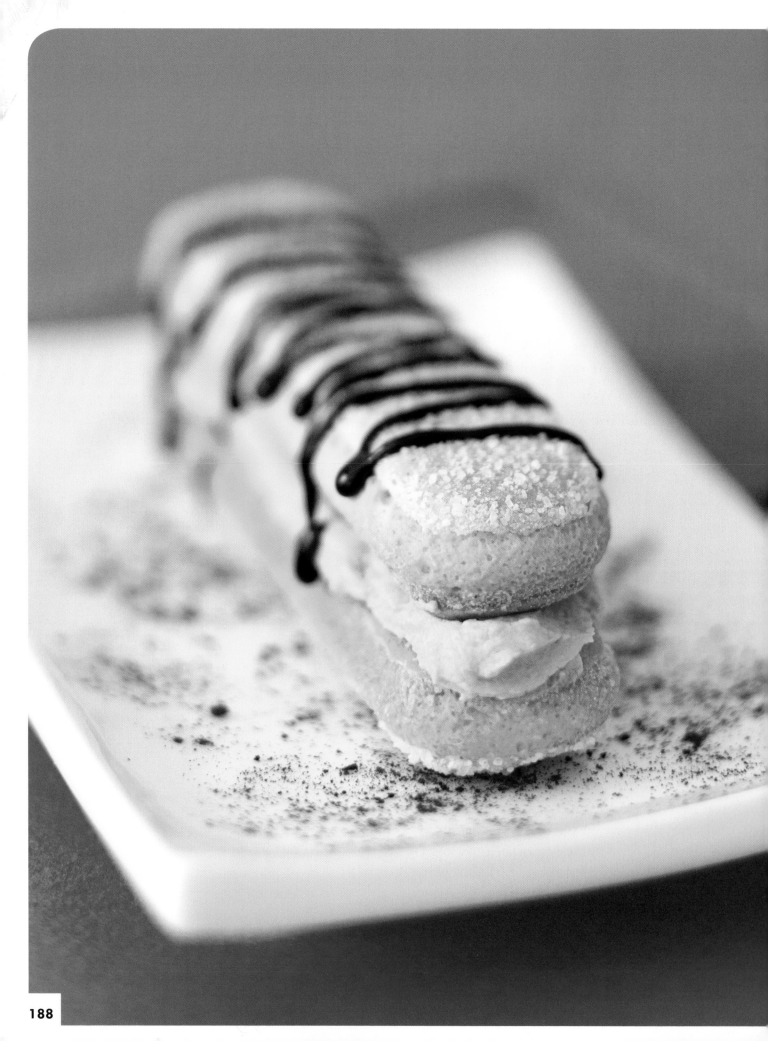

CALORIES	FAT	PROTEIN	CARBS	FIBER
135	3.5g	5g	21g	0g

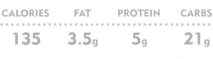

TIRAMISU PICK ME UPS

"These coffee-cream filled sandwich cookies are an evening pick-me-up that you can quite literally pick up with your bare hands… something I wouldn't recommend doing with traditional high-calorie tiramisu!"

YOU WILL NEED

1 (8-ounce) package fat-free cream cheese, softened

2 teaspoons instant coffee granules

2 ½ tablespoons sugar

½ teaspoon vanilla extract

24 ladyfinger cookies

¼ cup semi-sweet chocolate chips

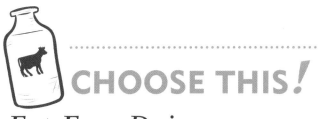

CHOOSE THIS!

Fat-Free Dairy, such as the fat-free cream cheese used in this recipe, can save you a ton of calories over their full-fat alternatives while still giving you most of the creaminess you are looking for. I find that using fat-free cream cheese in this recipe actually makes the filling smoother than regular cream cheese, which can be a little bit grainy.

1 Using a fork, cream together softened cream cheese, instant coffee, sugar, and vanilla extract until combined into a smooth and creamy filling.

2 Spread filling evenly over 12 of the ladyfinger cookies and then top each with a second cookie, sandwiching the filling inside.

3 In a microwave-safe bowl, microwave chocolate chips for 1 minute, stirring every 15 seconds, until entirely melted.

4 Drizzle melted chocolate over top each cookie sandwich. Refrigerate 15 minutes to set before serving.

THE SWEET STUFF

PREP TIME	COOK TIME	SERVES		CALORIES	FAT	PROTEIN	CARBS	FIBER
20 mins	10 mins	24		85	3.5g	1.5g	12.5g	2g

FRESH FRUIT PIZZA

"This dessert pizza is topped with a strawberry cream cheese 'sauce' and piled with an abundance of fresh and nutritious kiwi fruit, raspberries, blackberries, and blueberries."

YOU WILL NEED

nonstick cooking spray

1 (11-ounce) can thin pizza crust (such as Pillsbury)

1 (8-ounce) tub whipped strawberry cream cheese

2 kiwis, peeled and thinly sliced

1 pint raspberries

1 pint blackberries

1 pint blueberries

CHOOSE THIS!

Kiwis are absolutely bursting with immune system boosting vitamin C. In fact, you can get more than 100% of your daily recommended value of vitamin C in just one 50 calorie kiwi! Kiwis are also a good source of dietary fiber, potassium, magnesium, manganese, and vitamin E.

1 Preheat oven to 425 degrees F. Spray a sheet pan with nonstick cooking spray.

2 Unroll pizza dough onto the greased sheet pan and bake 8-10 minutes, until golden brown.

3 Remove crust from oven and let cool to room temperature before continuing.

4 Spread strawberry cream cheese over the entire surface of the cooled pizza crust and then top evenly with all fruit.

5 Slice into 24 pieces and serve room temperature. Note: I serve this with the crust room temperature, but I do like to chill the berries before topping.

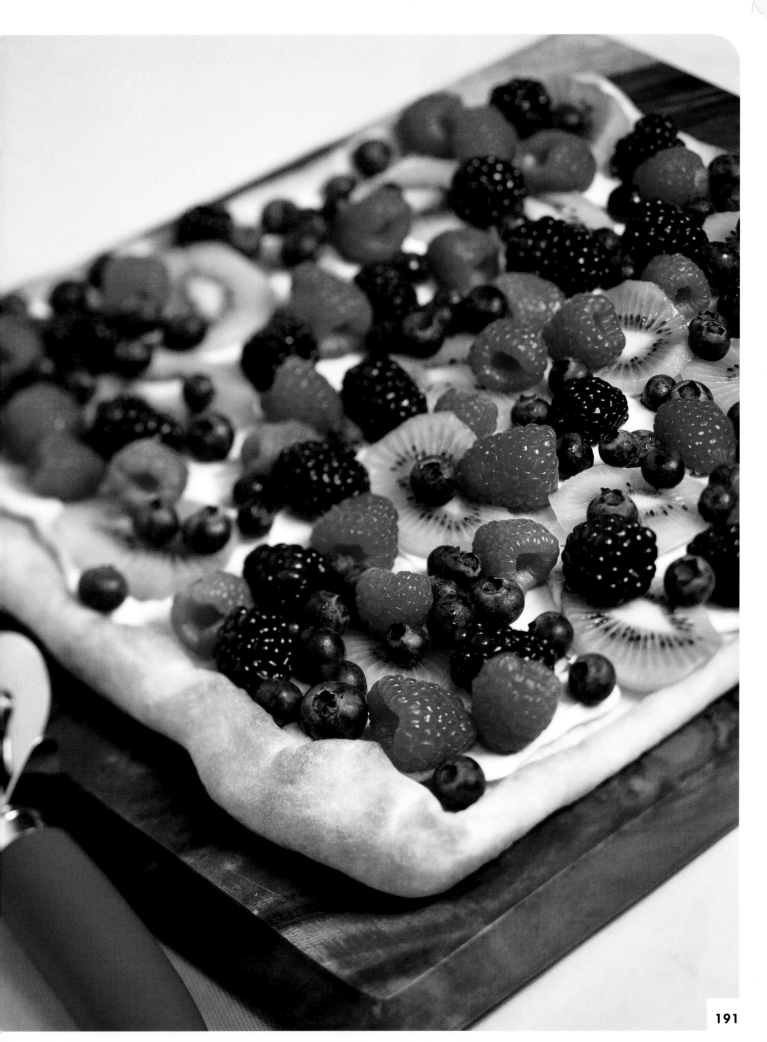

PREP TIME	COOK TIME	SERVES		CALORIES	FAT	PROTEIN	CARBS	FIBER
10 mins	varies	20		145	3g	3.5g	27g	2g

BETTER FOR YOU BROWNIES

"These types of brownies, made with puréed black beans in place of oil and eggs, have been around for a very long time and have always been my go-to way of preparing brownies. While I didn't come up with the idea (and can't find who actually did!), I must admit that they are genius! The only thing is that you can't tell anyone how you made them because they may pretend that they don't love these!"

YOU WILL NEED

nonstick cooking spray

1 (15-ounce) can black beans

1 (18.3-ounce) box brownie mix (for 13x9 pan)

½ cup chopped walnuts

CHOOSE THIS!

Black Beans, like most beans and legumes, are a very good source of fiber. Fiber can not only help aid in digestion and lower cholesterol but can also prevent blood sugar levels from rising too rapidly after meals.

1 Preheat oven to the temperature stated on the brownie mix box. Spray a 13x9 inch baking dish with nonstick cooking spray.

2 Drain and rinse black beans and then add back to the can that they came in. Fill the can, with beans still in it, to the very top with water.

3 Pour the beans and water into a food processor and purée until entirely smooth.

4 Mix puréed beans into the brownie mix until a smooth batter is created. Fold in walnuts.

5 Pour batter into the greased baking dish and bake according to the directions stated on the brownie mix box. (Slightly undercooked is fudgier!) Cut into 20 squares and serve warm or at room temperature.

PREP TIME	CHILL TIME	SERVES		CALORIES	FAT	PROTEIN	CARBS	FIBER
5 mins	30 mins	6		115	4.5g	1.5g	19g	1g

STRAWBERRY MOUSSE

"This simple strawberry mousse with only 115 calories per serving makes a really great dessert for entertaining guests when time is limited."

YOU WILL NEED

1 cup fat-free milk

1 (1.4-ounce) box vanilla instant pudding mix

1 cup frozen strawberries

1 (8-ounce) tub light non-dairy whipped topping

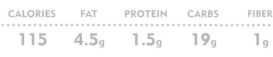

CHOOSE THIS!

Strawberries are filled with anthocyanins, which not only provide their flush red color but also serve as potent antioxidants that have been shown to help protect the body's cells from free-radical damage. This makes these delicious little berries a heart protecting, anti-inflammatory, and possibly even cancer preventing fruit all rolled into one.

1 Place milk and pudding mix into the bowl of a food processor.

2 Process pudding mixture for 30 seconds, until smooth and creamy.

3 Add strawberries to the mixture and pulse until roughly chopped before processing until entirely smooth, about 1 minute.

4 Using a rubber spatula, scrape mixture into a large mixing bowl and then gently fold in the non-dairy whipped topping, just until all is mostly combined. (A few swirls of white is just fine… in fact it looks quite nice!)

5 Cover and refrigerate for 30 minutes before spooning into parfait glasses to serve.

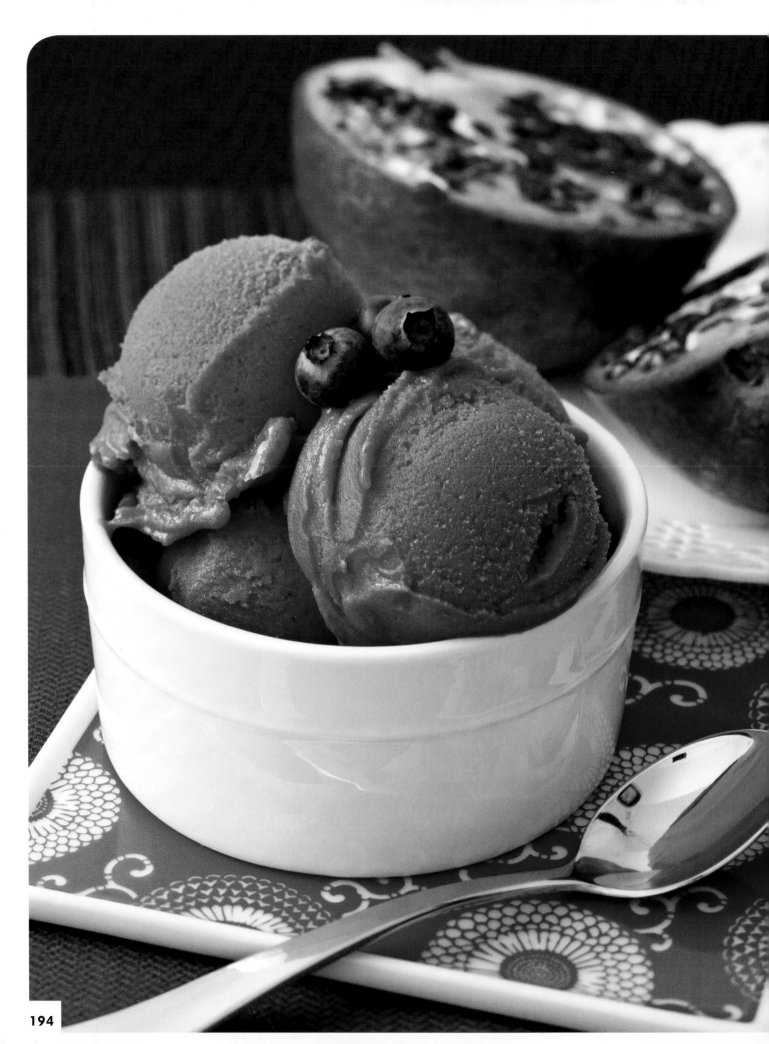

PREP TIME	CHILL TIME	SERVES		CALORIES	FAT	PROTEIN	CARBS	FIBER
15 mins	2 hrs	4		105	0g	1g	27g	3g

OH SO BERRY SORBET

"This sorbet is easily thrown together in only a few minutes and freezes into a nice, smooth consistency in just about 2 hours. Remember to save a few of the fresh berries for garnish!"

YOU WILL NEED

1 cup blueberries

1 cup strawberries

½ cup pomegranate juice

2 tablespoons lemon juice

¼ cup sugar

⅛ teaspoon salt

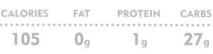

CHOOSE THIS!

The Berries in this sorbet—blueberries, strawberries, and pomegranates—not only make for an extremely refreshing sorbet, but they also pack it with a huge dose of antioxidants. It is quite possibly the most antioxidants per serving of any recipe in this book!

1 Place all ingredients into the bowl of a food processor or blender.

2 Process until entirely smooth, about 2 minutes.

3 Pour through a fine mesh strainer held over a freezer-safe container to catch any chunks of fruit that the processor left behind. (This step ensures the smoothest consistency but is entirely optional.)

4 Cover and freeze for at least 2 hours before serving. Let sit at room temperature for 5 minutes before serving for best consistency.

THE SWEET STUFF

PEACH CRISP CUPS

"I love peach cobblers and crisps, but they aren't exactly the most attractive or low-calorie dishes! This recipe solves both of those issues with conveniently portioned cups that are both elegant and relatively low in calories."

YOU WILL NEED

¼ cup brown sugar

¼ cup old-fashioned oats

½ teaspoon ground cinnamon

¼ teaspoon ground nutmeg

2 tablespoons butter, softened

2 tablespoons chopped pecans

2 peaches

CHOOSE THIS!

Peaches are a juicy and succulent source of beta-carotene, which not only gives them their peachy color, but also helps protect our eyes, heart, and other organs.

1 Preheat oven to 350 degrees F.

2 In a mixing bowl, combine brown sugar, oats, cinnamon, nutmeg, butter, and pecans to create a thick topping.

3 Gently rub peaches with a wet paper towel to remove most of their outer fuzz. Then, cut peaches in half and remove the pit.

4 Place each peach half, cut-side up, into individual baking dishes. Crumble an equal amount of the topping mixture over top of each.

5 Bake for 40-45 minutes, or until topping is golden brown. Serve warm.

PREP TIME	COOK TIME	SERVES		CALORIES	FAT	PROTEIN	CARBS	FIBER
15 mins	15 mins	24		160	6.5g	5g	21g	2.5g

HUNGER BUSTING PEANUT BUTTER COOKIES

"These nutty oatmeal cookies have a good amount of protein and fiber, which will ensure that you not only satisfy your sweet-tooth, but also keep it satisfied without the need to overeat!"

YOU WILL NEED

¾ cup nonfat plain yogurt

1 cup natural peanut butter

1 cup light brown sugar

1 large egg

2 teaspoons vanilla extract

1 cup whole wheat flour

2 ½ cups old-fashioned oats

1 teaspoon salt

1 ½ teaspoons ground cinnamon

2 teaspoons baking soda

CHOOSE THIS!

Peanuts (and the peanut butter used in this recipe) are a great source of mono-unsaturated fat and other nutrients shown to promote heart health. Natural peanut butter is best because it does not contain the added sugar, corn syrup, or oil that regular peanut butter can contain.

1 Preheat oven to 350 degrees F.

2 In a large mixing bowl, whisk together yogurt, peanut butter, and brown sugar. Add egg and vanilla extract, and continue whisking until combined.

3 In another mixing bowl, combine all remaining ingredients.

4 Add the dry ingredients to the wet ingredients, and stir until all is combined.

5 Spoon ¼ cup sized mounds of the dough onto cookie sheets, about 2 inches apart. Press each cookie down lightly to flatten.

6 Bake for 15 minutes before cooling on a wire rack at least 10 minutes. Serve slightly warm or at room temperature.

PREP TIME	COOK TIME	SERVES		CALORIES	FAT	PROTEIN	CARBS	FIBER
10 mins	none	1		210	11g	7g	23.5g	4g

RED, WHITE, AND BLUE YOGURT PARFAIT

"This patriotic parfait is bursting with fresh berry goodness. Sometimes the simplest things are the most delicious! Nutrition data is for 1 large parfait, but this could easily be split into 2 smaller glasses for 2 mini desserts."

YOU WILL NEED

½ cup strawberries, sliced

2 tablespoons chopped pecans

1 (6-ounce) container nonfat vanilla yogurt

¼ cup blueberries

1 pinch ground cinnamon

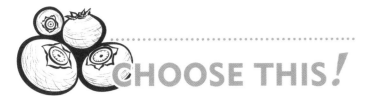

CHOOSE THIS!

Blueberries (as well as the strawberries in this recipe) are filled with anthocyanins that not only provide their color but also serve as potent antioxidants that have been shown to help protect the body's cells from free radical damage. This makes berries a heart protecting, anti-inflammatory, and possibly even cancer preventing fruit all rolled into one.

1 Place strawberries at the bottom of a tall and skinny parfait glass and sprinkle with a few of the chopped pecans.

2 Top with a layer of ½ of the yogurt, followed by another small sprinkle of the pecans.

3 Add all of the blueberries to create the third layer.

4 Add the remaining yogurt to create the fourth and final layer. Garnish the top with a small pinch of ground cinnamon, a few blueberries, and a slice of strawberry.

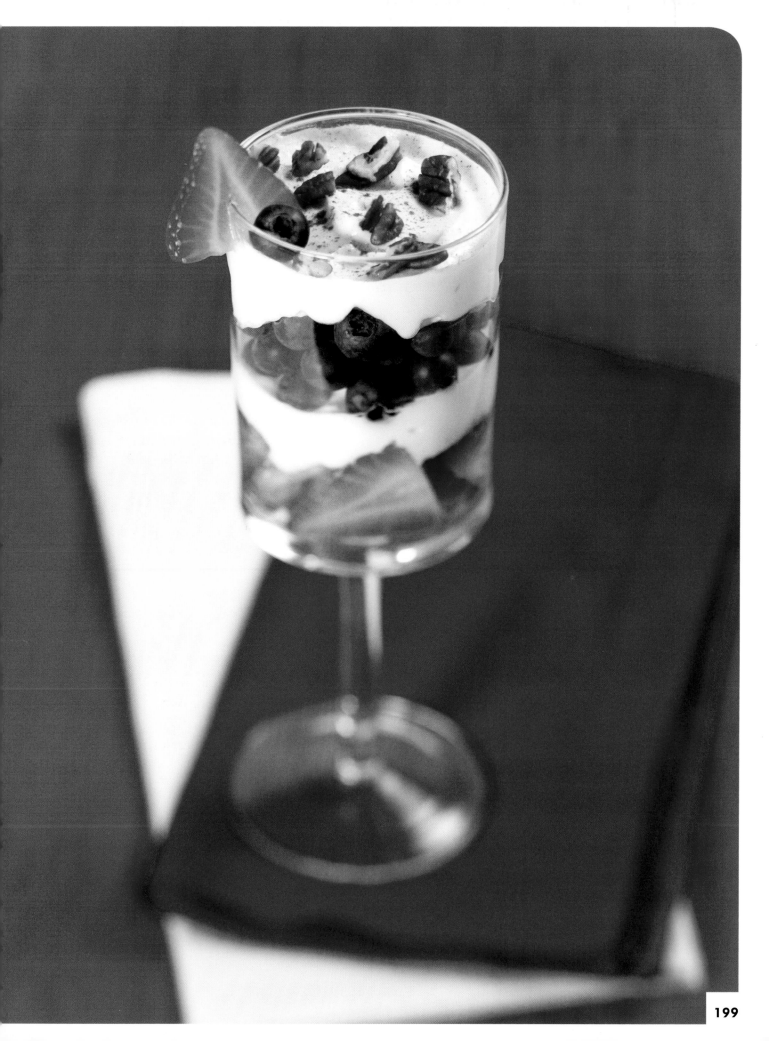

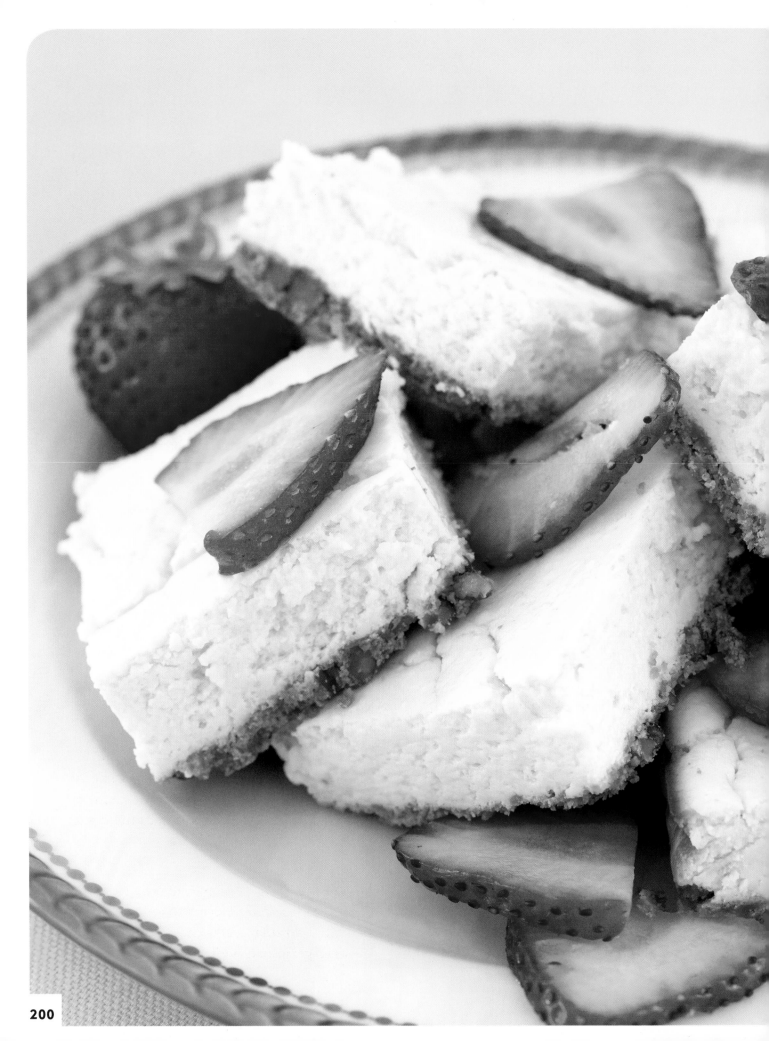

PREP TIME	COOK TIME	SERVES		CALORIES	FAT	PROTEIN	CARBS	FIBER
20 mins	40 mins	12		105	3g	7g	12g	0g

CHOOSE THESE CHEESECAKE SQUARES

"You would hardly believe that these luxurious cheesecake squares have only 3 grams of fat in each. That's as much as 20 times less fat than you'd get in a slice of restaurant cheesecake! With stats like that, choosing these couldn't be any easier."

YOU WILL NEED

nonstick cooking spray

½ cup graham cracker crumbs

¼ cup chopped pecans

1 tablespoon light butter, melted

2 (8-ounce) packages fat-free cream cheese, softened

3 large egg whites

¼ cup + 2 tablespoons sugar

2 teaspoons all-purpose flour

¾ teaspoon vanilla extract

½ teaspoon lemon juice

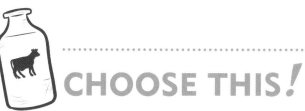

CHOOSE THIS!

Fat-Free Dairy, such as the fat-free cream cheese used in this recipe, can save you a ton of calories over their full-fat alternatives while still giving you most of the creaminess you are looking for. While fat-free cream cheese is not as solid as regular cream cheese, adding 2 teaspoons of flour to this recipe bulks it up quite well.

1 Preheat oven to 350 degrees F. Spray an 8x8 baking dish with nonstick cooking spray.

2 In a mixing bowl, combine graham cracker crumbs, chopped pecans, and melted butter, and then press down into the bottom of the baking dish to form a crust.

3 In an electric mixer, beat cream cheese, egg whites, all sugar, flour, vanilla extract, and lemon juice, just until ingredients are combined into a smooth cheesecake batter.

4 Spread cheesecake batter over the crust in the baking dish and bake 35-40 minutes, or until a toothpick inserted in the center comes out mostly clean.

5 Cool to room temperature on a wire rack before refrigerating at least 1 hour before serving. Slice into 12 squares and serve garnished with fresh fruit, if desired.

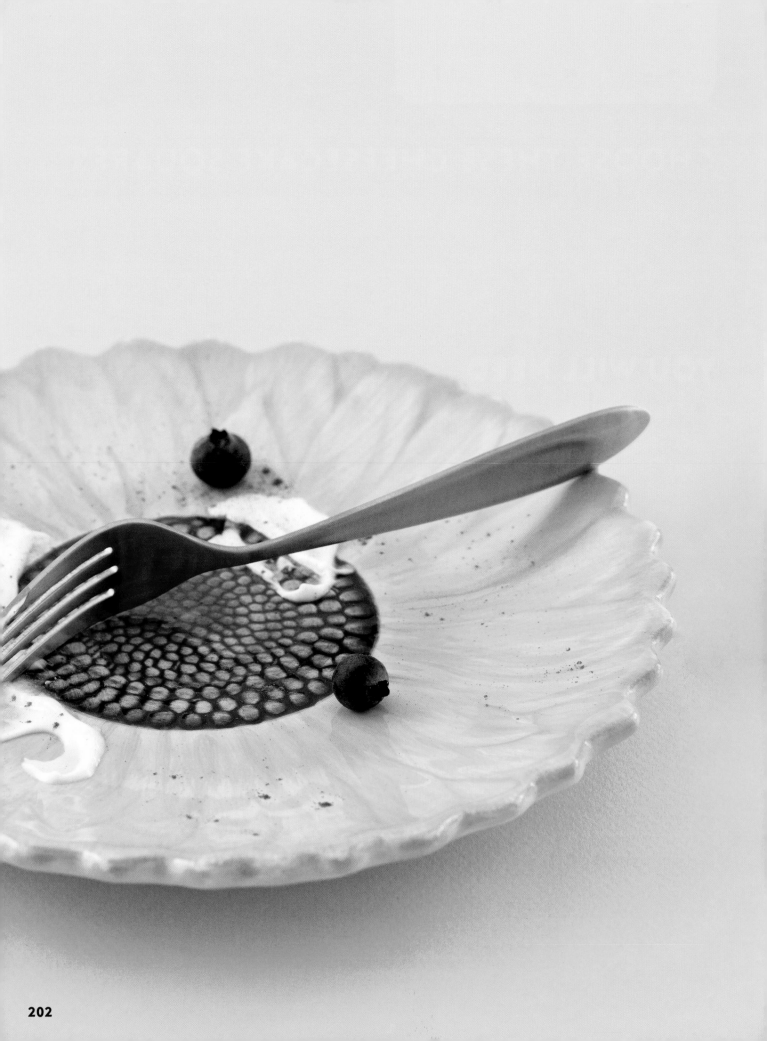

ABOUT THE AUTHOR

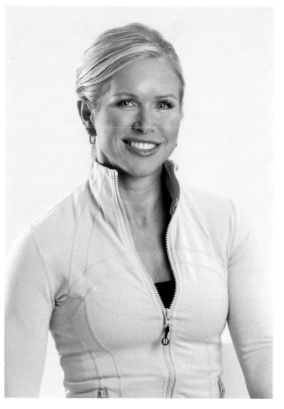

Chris Freytag

www.ChrisFreytag.com

Chris Freytag, a fitness professional and mother of three teenagers, understands firsthand the challenges of balancing healthy habits with the demands of a busy life. A contributing editor and columnist at Prevention magazine, she has also authored several books on fitness, weight loss, and healthy eating. She is a certified lifestyle and weight management coach, certified personal trainer, and sits on the board of directors for The American Council on Exercise. She readily admits that she has a sweet tooth and loves to eat.

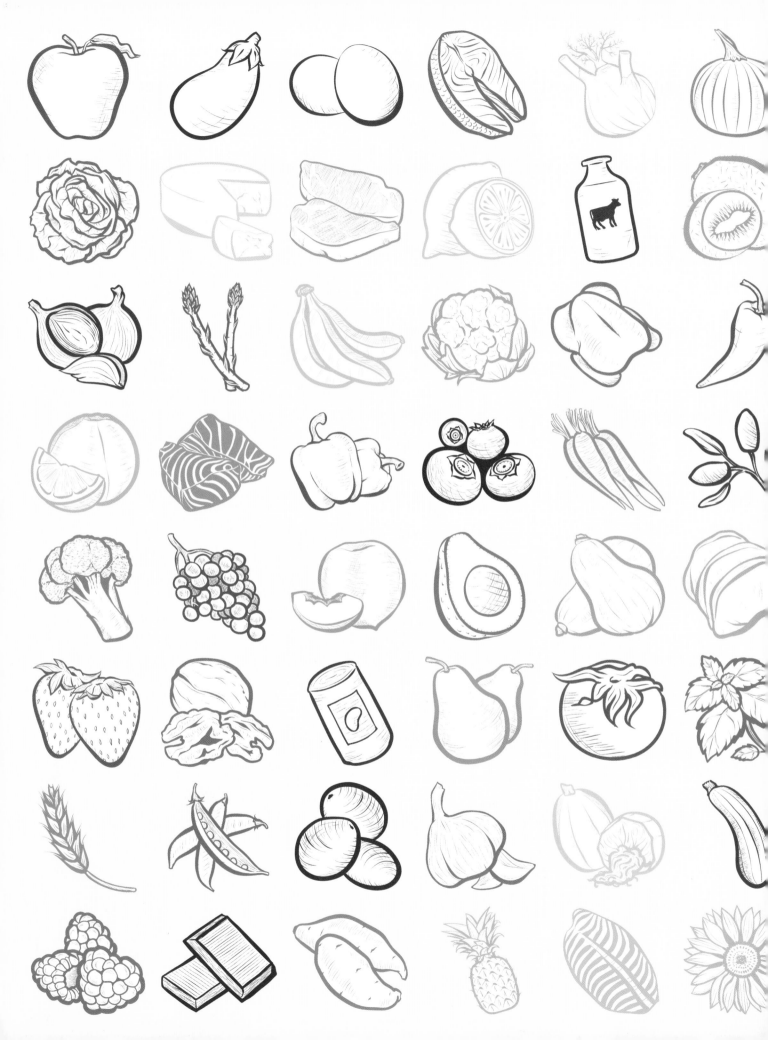

CHOOSE THESE INGREDIENTS!...........

Use this index to quickly recall the "Choose This!" information for all of the nutritious ingredients featured in this book.

RECIPE INDEX······

RECITE INDEX PAGE 2

RECIPE INDEX PAGE 3 ••••••••••••••••••••••••••••